Amyotrophic Lateral Sclerosis

Robert G. Miller, MD

Deborah Gelinas, MD

Patricia O'Connor, RN

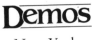

New York

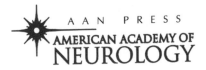

Demos Medical Publishing, 386 Park Avenue South, New York, NY 10016
www.demosmedpub.com

Library of Congress Cataloging-in-Publication Data

Miller, Robert G. (Robert Gordon), 1942–
　Amyotrophic lateral sclerosis / Robert G.Miller, Deborah Gelinas, Patricia O'Connor.
　　p. cm.
　Includes index.
　ISBN 1-932603-06-9 (pbk. : alk. paper)
　1.　Amyotrophic lateral sclerosis—Popular works.　I. Gelinas, Deborah F. (Deborah Faith), 1956–　II. O'Connor, Patricia, 1954–　III. Title.
　RC406.A24M556 2005
　616.8'3—dc22

2004018921

Contents

Section 3: Resources

Section 4: Appendix

Foreword

This book is one of the first in a series sponsored by the American Academy of Neurology designed to assist people with neurologic diseases and their families. This guide to amyotrophic lateral sclerosis, also known as *ALS* or *Lou Gehrig's disease*, appears at a propitious time for those confronted with newly diagnosed ALS, a particularly heart-rending disorder.

Hopes for prevention or cure have been raised by the accelerating pace of research in the past decade, starting with the discovery of a gene for familial ALS in 1993, followed within a year by the creation of an animal model in mice. We have gained more information about the cellular abnormalities in ALS from these mice than we did during the preceding 100 years. More scientists are working on the disease now than ever before. We know that before long, a cure or mode of prevention will protect us from this scourge. But we do not know how long it will take before that goal will be achieved, and patients need assistance now, not later.

The authors have wisely included informative chapters about the disease itself, specific symptoms and how they can be ameliorated, how multidisciplinary centers work, how voluntary health agencies help, how computers can help, how the Internet can be used, and even how to deal with the helter-skelter system of health insurance companies. These topics can guide patients to the best possible arrangement to meet their needs. The authors are all experts in the management of ALS, and this book will be much appreciated by patients and professionals alike.

Lewis P. Rowland, MD
Neurological Institute
Columbia University Medical Center
New York, NY

Acknowledgments

We wish to thank our patients and their families, whose courage in battling ALS inspired us to write this book.

We also wish to acknowledge the following members of the extraordinary multidisciplinary team of ALS specialists at the Forbes Norris MDA/ALS Research Center in San Francisco: Jodi Bales, Roberta Greenberg, Felicia Harte, Catherine Madison, Jason Mass, Sandy McDade, and Margie Petrakis. Each member of this team brings exceptional commitment, devotion, and clinical excellence to the care of our patients, and they have taught us much.

We are grateful to our own families who supported us during the writing of this book and were patient with us during our time taken away from family.

We wish to thank Ann Haugh for her considerable help with the graphic design of the figures and with the selection of the book cover, as well as help with the completion of the manuscripts. We also wish to thank Lois Esteban for her substantial help in completing the manuscripts.

We are most grateful for the superb chapters written by our contributors.

We wish to acknowledge the expertise and help of Dr. Diana M. Schneider, President of Demos Medical Publishing, for her review of the entire manuscript and support in producing this book.

We wish to acknowledge the tremendous contribution of Dr. Forbes Norris and Dee Holden Norris, RN, who worked tirelessly to raise the standard of care for patients with ALS. They too have inspired us to write this book.

Preface

If you are reading this book, we assume that you or a close family member or friend has been diagnosed with ALS, or that the diagnosis is under consideration. We have written this book to help you understand the disease and what can be done to manage it effectively.

ALS is a treatable disease, although it is far from being curable. We now have treatments that can make a major difference in enhancing the quality of life and prolonging life for those with this diagnosis. In addition, we have treatments for many of the symptoms of ALS that can help ease the burden of the disease. We have begun to use evidence-based medicine to select state-of-the-art management strategies for each and every patient with ALS. Multidisciplinary teams in specialized ALS centers provide top quality care and comprehensive rehabilitation for persons with ALS. The impact of various treatments for patients with ALS is now being measured in a continuing way using a North American patient database known as the *ALS CARE program*. ALS CARE is one of the first databases to track the outcome of this neurologic disease, thereby improving the standard of care for persons with ALS.

In spite of the progressive nature of ALS and its clear tendency to shorten life, there are a number of reasons for cautious optimism. One drug has been approved by regulatory agencies to slow the disease, albeit to a modest degree. As mentioned above, numerous other treatments are now available to help manage symptoms. The momentum of ALS research is expanding dramatically. Three new genes have been discovered in the last three years and numerous clinical trials are underway, testing promising new therapies. Both gene therapy and stem cell treatment have shown extremely promising results in animal models, and clinical trials in humans will hopefully start in the not too distant future. Our understanding of the basic causes of ALS is expanding gradually. The substantial resources of patient advocacy groups, such as the Muscular Dystrophy Association (MDA) and the Amyotrophic Lateral Sclerosis Association (ALSA), provide tremendous help and support for patients and families.

In spite of the adjustment required after learning that they have ALS, most patients tell us that life goes on. In fact, the vast majority of patients begin living life again fully and with joy and courage after working through the initial transition and adjustment to the diagnosis. Many of our patients become extraordinary heroes and discover new courage from within to battle the disease and live life with vigor and enthusiasm. It is our sincere hope that the information in this book will prove useful to you in proactively managing your ALS.

The book begins with a discussion of the nature of the disease process in ALS, how symptoms develop, how the disease is diagnosed, and the therapies available to slow its progress. We then discuss treating the symptoms of ALS and the benefits of receiving care in a specialized ALS center, emphasizing the importance of preserving quality of life and addressing family and social issues. Chapters on nutrition, communication, getting around and staying active, sleeping and breathing issues, and the changes in personality and thinking that affect some people with ALS will help readers to better cope with these aspects of the disease process. A consideration of end-of-life issues emphasizes approaching the advanced stages of ALS with dignity. Finally, a summary of helpful resources is provided to help ease the burden of the disease.

Robert G. Miller, MD
Deborah Gelinas, MD
Patricia O'Connor, RN

Authors

Robert G. Miller, M.D.
Director
Forbes Norris MDA/ALS Research Center
Chairman, Dept. of Neurosciences
California Pacific Medical Center
San Francisco, California

Deborah F. Gelinas, MD
Clinical Director
Forbes Norris MDA/ALS Research Center
California Pacific Medical Center
San Francisco, California

Patricia O'Connor, RN
Nurse Case Manager
Forbes Norris MDA/ALS Research Center
California Pacific Medical Center
San Francisco, California

With contributions by:
Alycia Chu, MS, RD
Nutritionist
Forbes Norris MDA/ALS Research Center
California Pacific Medical Center
San Francisco, California

Susan Woolley Levine, PhD
Clinical Psychologist
Forbes Norris MDA/ALS Research Center
California Pacific Medical Center
San Francisco, California

Mary Lyon, RN, MN
Vice President, Patient Services
ALS Association
Calabasas Hills, California

Amy Roman, MS, CCC-SLP
Speech Therapist
Forbes Norris MDA/ALS Research Center
California Pacific Medical Center
San Francisco, California

Ronald J. Schenkenberger, BS
Director of Research Administration
Muscular Dystrophy Association
Tucson, Arizona

Dorothy E. Northrop, MSW, ACSW
Director of Clinical Programs
National Multiple Sclerosis Society
New York, New York

SECTION I

Introduction

CHAPTER 1

What Is Amyotrophic Lateral Sclerosis?

Amyotrophic lateral sclerosis (ALS) results from degeneration of the *motor nerve cells* (or motor neurons) in the brain and spinal cord. These are the nerve cells that control the muscles (see Figure 1-1) Muscular weakness develops as the disease progresses and the nerves become more affected by the disease process. This weakness may appear in the legs, the arms, or in the muscles used for speech, swallowing, or breathing. The various symptoms that people experience when they have ALS are discussed in much more detail below.

ALS is considered by many experts to be a member of a family of neurologic diseases. The motor neurons begin to degenerate and stop functioning in people with ALS, which leads to progressive weakness. A similar thing happens to people who have Alzheimer's disease, in which the cells responsible for memory and thinking begin to deteriorate. In Parkinson's disease, the nerve cells that control the coordination of the body stop functioning properly and deteriorate. These diseases all have one thing in common: a certain type of nerve cell begins to degenerate and gradually and steadily causes increasing disease. Research suggests that there are common factors in all of these *neurodegenerative diseases* that may be important and that might suggest targets for therapy. Research along these lines is accelerating and beginning to look very promising.

What's in a Name?

ALS is often referred to as *Lou Gehrig's disease*. The world-renowned baseball player for the New York Yankees is probably the most famous individual who ever developed ALS. His record for the most consecutive

3

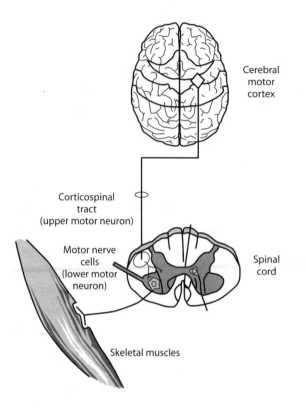

FIGURE 1-1

Upper and lower motor neuron connections between the brain and muscle.

baseball games played by any baseball player stood for 60 years. He is a symbol of determination and courage in the struggle against ALS, and his famous quote, "I am the luckiest man alive," when he retired from pro-

ALS is often referred to as *Lou Gehrig's disease.*

fessional baseball because of progressive weakness, is still regarded as a study in heroism.

Other terms are frequently utilized to describe ALS and related conditions. The term *motor neuron disease* (MND) refers to any condition that causes progressive weakening of the muscles as a result of the loss of motor nerve cells. This broad term encompasses a number of other diseases, such as postpolio syndrome and spinal muscular atrophy. ALS is a type of motor neuron disease. *Progressive muscular atrophy* is a term utilized by many physicians to refer to progressive weakness and thinning of the muscles when the diagnosis of ALS cannot be made. For people who have progressive muscular atrophy, the criteria for the diagnosis of ALS are not fulfilled. This is considered a hopeful situation and possibly a more benign condition than ALS. *Primary lateral sclerosis* is another condition that involves degeneration of motor neurons, causing clumsiness, stiffness, and awkwardness, as well as slowness—as opposed to weakness and thinning of muscles. This condition also is more slowly progressive than ALS and generally considered to be more benign. Some of the technical differences between these different conditions will be discussed later. *Bulbar palsy* and *pseudobulbar palsy* are terms that describe the impairment of the muscular function involved in speech and swallowing. These terms are often used to indicate a localized motor neuron abnormality when the speech and swallowing muscles are the only ones affected. The majority of people with progressive muscular atrophy, primary lateral sclerosis, bulbar palsy, or pseudobulbar palsy do, later on, fulfill criteria for the diagnosis of ALS. However, there are notable exceptions to this general rule and a significant number of patients stay in the more benign categories.

The term *amyotrophic lateral sclerosis* is of Greek origin. The phrase *myo* refers to the muscle; *a* means a negative impact on the muscle; and *trophic* indicates the decreasing nutrition of the muscle. Thus, *amyotrophic* refers to the thinning and wasting of the muscles. This muscle thinning is often referred to as *atrophy* or *amyotrophy*. The word *lateral* refers to the location of the nerve cells that deteriorate in the spinal cord, which are located on its far edge. These nerve cells are like telephone cables that connect the brain with the nerve cells that directly transmit impulses to muscles. When these nerve cells degenerate and die, they leave a scar in the spinal cord that is referred to as *sclerosis*, the last part of the name for ALS.

Why Does Someone Develop ALS?

ALS is considered a rare disease because only two people out of 100,000 in the general population develop it. Surprisingly, the frequency of occurrence of new cases of ALS is similar to that of new cases of multiple scle-

5

rosis (MS), which is probably better recognized and more familiar to more people. Approximately 10,000 new cases of both diseases appear each year

> Current estimates are that between 20,000 and
> 30,000 Americans are living with ALS.

in the United States. Current estimates are that between 20,000 and 30,000 Americans are living with ALS. The age of disease onset is highly variable, with an average in the late 50s but with a broad span from the early 20s to the 90s. The majority of patients first develop symptoms between the ages of 40 and 70, but many younger and older patients exist.

We do not know why certain people develop ALS, but we do know that the disease is more common in men than women by a ratio of 3:2. We also know that men tend to develop the disease at a younger age than women. These factors suggest that women may be somewhat protected from developing ALS, but the reasons for this are still unclear.

The biggest breakthrough in the field of ALS was the discovery in 1993 of a gene that is linked to the development of the disease. This gene coordinates the manufacture of a specific protein called *superoxide dismutase 1 (SOD-1)*, whose function is to clean the cell of the waste products of cell metabolism known as *free radicals*. (When a gene is abnormal, the protein that it produces does not function normally, and the functions that the protein controls will also be affected.) Detailed discussion of the function of the abnormal enzyme in people with this gene who develop ALS will be provided in more detail in later chapters.

Five to ten percent of people with ALS have a clear-cut pattern of the disease, often over several generations of their families. Of these patients with a clear family history of ALS, 20 percent have the abnormal SOD-1 gene. People who have this gene are considered to have a *familial* type of ALS, even though the majority of people with familial ALS (80 percent) do not carry the abnormal SOD-1 gene. People with the SOD-1 gene abnormality (known as a *mutation* or disturbance in the gene) can inherit it from either parent. This gene is a strong gene having an *autosomal dominant* characteristic. Thus, each child who has an affected parent who is known to carry the gene has a 50 percent chance of inheriting the abnormal gene and developing ALS. In virtually all people who have the gene, there is a strong family history of ALS. Typically, a person who develops familial ALS had a mother or father with the disease, and a grandparent who had the disease; usually there are also numerous other affected family members.

Because 90 to 95 percent of people with ALS do not have a family history of the disease, and only 20 percent of those with a family history have the SOD-1 gene abnormality, only 1 to 2 percent of people with ALS actually have the SOD-1 gene abnormality. Routine testing for the SOD-1 gene has become available through commercial laboratories, but it is not recommended in the vast majority of patients because of the very low sensitivity of the test: 98 to 99 percent of people will be negative on the SOD-1 gene test even though they have ALS.

Thus, a person with ALS who has a family history of ALS (especially a sibling or parent) probably inherited a gene that is sometimes a SOD-1 abnormality but, more often, it is a gene that we cannot yet measure. In the other 90 or 95 percent of people for whom there is no family history, the reason for developing ALS is still unclear. In patients without a family history of ALS, the chances of passing the disease on to their children are extremely rare.

There are other causes of ALS besides an abnormal gene. One of the most popular theories relates to the excessive stimulation of motor nerve cells by a substance known as *glutamate*. This is a compound that exists normally throughout the brain and spinal cord. It is necessary for nerve cells to communicate with one another, and also for normal growth and metabolism. Nerve cells cannot "speak" with one another without glutamate; however, excessive amounts of glutamate can be distinctly harmful to nerve cells. There is evidence in ALS to suggest that glutamate builds up in the strategic areas of the brain and spinal cord where motor neurons are located, and that too much glutamate contributes to the damage of the motor neurons. The only approved drug available for slowing down the disease process in ALS is riluzole (Rilutek®), which interferes with the build-up of glutamate and delays the progress of the disease. This is an area of intense current research to find more effective therapies.

The build-up of abnormal products of metabolism is another area of current research interest. The discovery of the SOD-1 gene mutation has led to an explosion in research on the build-up of toxic waste products within the cell. Oxidized substances accumulate in all cells as a result of their normal energy requirements and processes. In many ways, the build-up of such waste products is similar to what happens when metal is left out in the rain and begins to rust. Rust is a build-up of products that are referred to as *oxidative*; they are related to excessive oxygen product accumulation. These toxic products are known as *free radicals* or *reactive oxygen species*. Antioxidants such as vitamin E may reduce the excessive accumulation of this type of toxic waste product in human cells.

Another area of great excitement in the search for the cause of ALS is the role of inflammation within the brain and spinal cord. Emerging evidence suggests that excessive inflammation occurs within the nerve cells in the motor control regions of people with ALS. Some investigators believe that the body's immune system becomes activated and misdirected in ALS, producing some of the abnormalities that are important in developing the disease. Clinical trials are under way to explore the therapeutic benefit of anti-inflammatory drugs in ALS, which is discussed in more detail in later chapters.

All of these harmful substances—glutamate excitotoxicity, oxidative stress, and inflammation—damage the motor neuron. As injury to the nerve cell worsens, it moves to a final common pathway of *apoptosis*, or *preprogrammed cell death*. New agents that block apoptosis are emerging, and a few (minocycline and a new Novartis agent called *TCH346*) are under investigation in human clinical trials.

A number of studies have shown that certain factors are more common in people with ALS than in people who do not have the disease. A history of smoking appears to place a person at increased risk for the disease. The risk is proportional to the amount of smoking, the number of years of smoking, and whether a person is still smoking. Some studies suggest that prior injuries or trauma may predispose one to ALS, and others suggest that people who are athletic and engage in competitive sports may be at increased risk. There is one report of an increase of ALS in veterans who served in the Gulf War. There is still no clear understanding of this association, although some toxin exposure is suspected; but many of these factors are not well understood in terms of their role in producing ALS. The role of viruses and exposure to heavy metals and other toxins has been investigated with mixed results. At the present time, there is no compelling evidence that a virus or a toxin is involved with ALS, but these are areas that deserve further research.

What Are Some of the Early Symptoms of ALS?

The initial sign of ALS for most people is the development of localized weakness in one area of the body. It may begin in a foot or hand, an arm

> The initial sign of ALS for most people is the development of localized weakness in one area of the body.

or leg, the speech or swallowing muscles, or even, rarely, the breathing muscles. The muscles may become weak and thin in the affected area, or they may become slow and awkward. Weakness usually becomes more obvious and more marked with time.

Weakness and thinning (*atrophy*) of the muscles indicate abnormalities in those cells of the nervous system called *lower motor neurons* (see Figure 1-1). Lower motor neurons are the nerve cells that carry messages from the spinal cord to the muscles. They are a major target of the disease. When the lower motor neurons are abnormal, the muscles that they innervate become weakened and thinned. As noted above, this usually begins in one part of the body, such as a foot or a hand, although occasionally the weakness may be noticeable in more than one part of the body at the beginning. There is a tendency for the weakness to begin and to remain localized in one part of the body for some period of time before spreading to another part. Common early symptoms are foot slapping when there is foot and ankle weakness, or difficulty opening jars or turning keys when there is hand weakness. Slurring of speech or slowing of speaking is also an early sign in some people.

The symptoms of ALS are different when the disease initially affects the *upper motor neurons* (see Figure 1-1). Upper motor neurons are the connections between the brain and the lower motor neurons in the spinal cord. When you reach out to shake someone's hand, the signal originates at the top of the brain surface and travels through the upper motor neuron down into the spinal cord. Within the spinal cord, it passes the signal to a lower motor neuron, which then exits the spinal cord and travels through the limb to your hand, where it activates the muscles to carry out the desired act. When upper motor neurons are disturbed, as they commonly are in ALS, the hand will not function automatically and quickly. Awkwardness, clumsiness, and slowness of hand function result from upper motor neuron dysfunction affecting the nerves that control the hand. Stiffness and slowness, and awkwardness of the leg or foot result from impairment of the upper motor neuron that governs leg and foot control. Slow, slurred speech is an indication that the upper motor neurons controlling speech and swallowing have been affected.

The progressive impairment of muscle control in ALS causes symptoms to worsen steadily over time. The speed of worsening is widely variable from person to person, an important factor that we will return to at the end of this chapter. In ALS, simultaneous involvement of both the upper and the lower motor neurons is usually seen. Thus, most patients develop both weakness and thinning of muscles, as well as stiffness and slowing of muscle control. The terms *bulbar* and *pseudobulbar*, as discussed previously, are also important terms to be familiar with because health care professionals often use these terms. The bulbar muscles are those that are important in speech and swallowing. A lower motor neuron abnormality that affects the bulbar muscles will result in slurred speech and difficulty in swallowing. This is called *bulbar palsy*. An upper motor neuron abnormality that affects the speech and swallowing muscles is called *pseudobulbar palsy*. This kind of dysfunction results in slow, slurred speech and also in increased emotionality. Another term for the increased emotionality of ALS is *emotional incontinence*, which refers to the tendency of people with this problem to laugh or cry excessively even though they may not feel happy or sad at the time. This unusual symptom is very bothersome and embarrassing to patients, and very troubling and frustrating for families. It can be effectively treated with a number of widely available medications. Therapy for these various problems is discussed extensively in later chapters.

Very occasionally, the first symptom of ALS is difficulty in breathing. This occurs when the nerves that nourish and control the muscles involved in breathing are selectively affected early in the course of the disease. People may find themselves becoming short of breath with exertion, or even experience difficulty with breathing while sitting or lying. Effective treatment for breathing difficulties is available to help manage this very serious and troublesome symptom of ALS, and will be discussed in detail in a later chapter.

Weight loss is very common in ALS and may result from muscle thinning and muscle loss, as well as from reduced caloric intake. Some people become depressed and lose their appetite when they have ALS. Others who have swallowing difficulties may not take in enough calories to meet the energy demands of the body. There is evidence that the energy metabolism of the body is somewhat accelerated in people with ALS, so that increased caloric intake is often necessary to maintain weight. A number of effective treatments are available to maintain weight and prevent malnutrition, which may exaggerate the fatigue and weakness, and accelerate the disease process.

Muscle cramps are a common early symptom in people with ALS. The precise cause of the cramps is not entirely clear, but the abnormality of the motor nerves is an important ingredient in the excessive cramping. Cramps often occur in areas of muscular weakness and muscle thinning. Treatment for muscle cramps is often effective, as discussed below.

Muscle twitching is present in almost all patients with ALS. These twitches are called *fasciculations*. Often, the person with ALS is not aware he or she is twitching until it is pointed out by a loved one or health care professional. Fasciculations occur in people without ALS as well. For example, all of us have twitching in our muscles after heavy exercise or under periods of stress, anxiety, or fatigue. However, they are more common and more frequent in ALS. When ALS patients become aware of them, they may become preoccupied with the twitching and assume that it is a bad sign of progressing disease. In fact, fasciculations have *no* clinical significance with respect to disease progression. There is no effective treatment for fasciculations, nor is treatment needed because they are not painful. The best advice that we can give about fasciculations is to ignore them.

What Treatments Are Available for ALS?

Until relatively recently, ALS was considered an untreatable disease. The truth is that ALS is a treatable disease even though it is not curable. One drug has been approved by the Food and Drug Administration to slow the

> ALS is a treatable disease even though it is not curable.

disease progression: riluzole (Rilutek®). Much more will be said about this drug in later chapters. Treatment is available to maintain normal nutrition, and for abnormal breathing, cramps, difficulty with mobility, excessive emotionality, depression, fatigue, stiffness, bladder difficulty, and sleeping difficulties. Thus, ALS is a treatable disease that is best treated by experts who are experienced and familiar with its many manifestations. The multidisciplinary teams available in large ALS centers provide an incredible breadth and depth of resources to help manage the disease. These teams of experts usually include a neurologist, nurse, social worker, physical therapist, occupational therapist, nutritionist, speech therapist, psychologist, and a patient advocacy representative. Much more will be said about multidisciplinary treatment in subsequent chapters. The important thing to remember is that ALS is a treatable disease even though it is not curable.

What Does the Future Hold for Someone with ALS?

ALS is a progressive disease, but its rate of progression is different for every individual. There are malignant forms of the disease in which the affected person may die less than a year after onset. Fortunately, these are rare. By contrast, there have been a few instances in which patients have completely recovered from ALS, although these cases are also very rare. Most patients survive 3 to 5 years after onset of the disease, but fully 20 percent of patients

> ALS is a progressive disease, but its rate of progression is different for every individual.

will beat these odds. In fact, 10 percent of patients will live more than 10 years with the disease and still have quality in their lives. The factors that seem to correlate with slow progression and a more favorable outcome include: younger age of onset; onset in the limbs rather than in the speech, swallowing, or breathing muscles; a long interval between the onset of symptoms and establishing a diagnosis; the presence of a marital or close supportive partner; a network of supportive friends and family; a positive attitude; a strong sense of spirituality; and a self-perception of good quality of life in the affected individual. Contrary to popular belief, all of us who work in the field have experience with individuals who struggle successfully with ALS over 20 to 25 years and still have real quality in their lives. Moreover, although most people go through a period of depression and appropriate sadness when initially coming to grips with the diagnosis, the vast majority of them adapt to the disease and resume a healthy and meaningful lifestyle. Quality of life can only be assessed by the person with ALS. Studies show that other people may underestimate a person's quality of life compared to that person's own rating of his quality of life. What is most important is an individuals' attitude and feeling about their own quality of life.

Reasons to Be Hopeful

Most people are in shock when they first hear that they have ALS. The diagnosis of ALS is admittedly one of the most devastating that we can imagine. We have worked with thousands of patients with ALS and can attest to the fact that—in spite of the burden of dealing with this disease—there are still reasons to be hopeful.

The first reason to be hopeful is that there is life after the diagnosis of ALS. People go through a transition period that includes a substantial amount of anger and grieving when they first hear the diagnosis. Then, often in an extraordinary way, people get beyond this initial reaction and begin living their lives again even more fully than before. Many patients have said to us that their lives took on new meaning and richness after they came to grips with the diagnosis.

Second, there has been an explosion in research in this field. The number of new laboratories investigating ALS has risen in an astronomical fashion over the last five years. With the discovery of an increasing number of genes and new potential therapies for ALS, the future is bright. Stem cells and gene therapy hold extraordinary promise.

Third, numerous clinical trials are under way, and participating in a clinical trial has tremendous advantages for the person with ALS. Participants in clinical trials make a contribution to further our understanding of the disease and possibly to finding new treatments. In addition, they may receive a treatment that will prove to be beneficial in slowing the disease process. Participating in a clinical trial engenders hope and provides an additional dimension to fighting the disease. Participants have their finger on the pulse of what's new; they are at the cutting edge of research in ALS.

Fourth, the treatments available for the many symptoms of ALS have expanded dramatically in the last five years. ALS is now truly a treatable disease with many symptomatic therapies that ease its burden and facilitate its management.

CHAPTER 2

The Diagnosis of ALS

A tremendous amount of anxiety surrounds the diagnosis of ALS. There is considerable fear on the part of patients and families in hearing the diagnosis, and there may be a considerable degree of denial and wishing to avoid hearing the diagnosis. There is also an understandable reluctance to give the diagnosis on the part of physicians, who may defer telling the bad news until there is absolutely no remaining doubt about the diagnosis. These factors partly explain the delay in the diagnosis of ALS, which often exceeds one year from the time of symptom onset. These sources of delay may, in fact, interfere with therapeutic intervention that might make a real difference in terms of both quality and length of life. There are arguments both for and against early diagnosis. We will address these issues in this chapter and talk about how the diagnosis is made and what confounding factors can sometimes make it difficult to render an earlier definite diagnosis.

Understanding the complexity of establishing the diagnosis of ALS is often helpful for patients and families. At the present time, there is no single test that can establish the diagnosis with certainty, and there are a number of tests that should be considered to rule out a condition that might mimic ALS. This chapter reviews the process through which a diagnosis of ALS is made.

Telling the Story

Every person with ALS has a different experience with the disease. Some people experience a slow gradual development of weakness in one part of the body, while for others, the symptoms appear to come on very rapidly. For most people, the first definite symptom of the disease is weakness appearing in one arm or leg, but occasionally speech and swallowing or even breathing muscles are affected first. Many people gradually accommodate to the subtle onset of weakness and may wait for extended time intervals before seeking medical attention. Some people may have symptoms for only a few weeks prior to seeking medical attention and, in general, this tends to suggest a more rapid progress of the disease. Still others do not notice symptoms and do not seek medical advice for months and even years, suggesting a more slowly progressive type of ALS. Some people have surgery because of the suspicion of a pinched nerve in the neck, back, or even in the limbs (such as for carpal tunnel syndrome). Sometimes there is even temporary improvement after surgery, which suggests a diagnosis other than ALS. In true ALS, however, patients continue to worsen after surgery and it becomes clear over time that a progressive disease is present rather than a pinched nerve.

The neurologist will generally want to listen to the whole story about how your symptoms developed. This will usually be followed by a series of questions designed to elaborate the symptoms in greater detail. Symptoms of weakness in the hand may lead to trouble opening jars, turning keys, or opening doors, and these will be analyzed in some detail. The same is true for symptoms involving the legs and whether there are difficulties going up and down stairs, catching the toe, having the ankle roll over on uneven ground, or difficulty rising from a chair. Symptoms involving the legs may also include knees buckling or falling. A series of questions will also focus on speech and swallowing and whether there has been any choking or reduction in caloric intake as a result of any swallowing difficulty. Any excessive emotionality—either laughter or crying—that is difficult to control should be reported; this is a common symptom in people with ALS. There will be questions about breathing because of the importance of the strength of the muscles for breathing in determining longevity in ALS.

Some patients with ALS may develop sensory symptoms such as heaviness or coldness and, rarely, even numbness or tingling in the hands or feet. When these symptoms are prominent, it tends to raise questions about the accuracy of the diagnosis. Similarly, questions about bladder and bowel function are mainly designed to rule out other neurologic conditions, because bladder and bowel function are usually unaffected until later in the course of the disease. Memory and thinking function are also generally spared in people with ALS, although subtle changes in personality and behavior have been reported. Occasional patients with ALS may have memory loss, so there will usually be questions along these lines as well. Pain, while not uncommon in the advanced stages of the disease, is generally quite unusual in the early stages of ALS and would also raise a question about the diagnosis.

Questions about general health are also relevant to determine whether a systemic disease might explain some of the symptoms. For example, patients who have cancer may have symptoms of weakness and fatigue, and patients with hormone disturbances including the thyroid or

> The existence of a family member with ALS is an important part of an individual's history.

parathyroid gland may also have similar symptoms. Exposure to toxic materials, such as lead, mercury, or arsenic, might produce some of the symptoms of ALS; the same is true for exposure to some infectious diseases, such as Lyme disease.

The existence of a family member with ALS is an important part of an individual's history. A family history of ALS in a person with the symptoms of ALS strongly supports the diagnosis. Sometimes, however, family members have nonspecific symptoms that are not indicative of ALS but that do indicate how fearful and anxious family members can become. The following vignette illustrates this issue:

A 35-year-old woman complained of generalized fatigue and muscle twitching of 6-months' duration. Her father had died of ALS one year previously. A comprehensive evaluation disclosed no abnormality of nerve or muscle function and no evidence of ALS. In spite of reassurance, she was unable to shake the fear of having ALS. Over the next 18 months, with counseling, antidepressant medication, and continued normal follow-up exam-

inations, she finally realized that her fatigue had been caused by depression and worry, not ALS.

Comment: *This scenario, in which the loss of a family member from ALS engenders fear in other family members and friends, is not uncommon. Health care providers are also susceptible to this kind of fear and worry, and may overreact to cramps, twitches, or fatigue as possibly indicating ALS. Fortunately, the opinion of an expert in ALS is sufficient reassurance for most people that they do not have the disease.*

The neurologist should also be told about symptoms of emotional upheaval. When a diagnosis of ALS is being considered, many people become depressed or anxious, have a disrupted sleep pattern, and feel tremendous fatigue because of the stress related to the possible diagnosis. The neurologist can often help in managing these symptoms.

The Neurologic Examination

The neurologist is trained to detect abnormalities during a physical examination that suggest an underlying disease of the nervous system. The neurologic examination includes having a look at the entire body to see if muscles are twitching or becoming thin. An examination of intellectual function and memory is also carried out to ensure that there is no impairment in these areas. If a person is extremely worried, stressed, or anxious, it may be difficult to function normally on this type of test. However, clear-cut abnormalities of thought processes may point to the presence of some condition other than ALS.

The muscles of speech and swallowing are tested thoroughly during the examination to search for subtle abnormalities. The tongue is inspected for muscle bulk and the presence of twitching as well as muscle weakness. The same is true for the other muscles of speech and swallowing in the mouth and palate. Difficulty pronouncing and articulating words points to a defect in the motor control of these muscles for speech. Excessive crying or laughter during the examination also supports the diagnosis of ALS. Some people are unable to resist crying even when there is no feeling of sadness; the crying may be prolonged and difficult to stop. The same is true (although less common) for outbreaks of laughter that may be inappropriate. These symptoms are common in people with ALS who have difficulties with speech and swallowing. Other functions in this part of the examination include vision, hearing, and smell, which are usually completely normal in persons with ALS.

The limbs are then examined for signs of weakness, thinning, and twitching, which indicate that a *lower motor neuron* disturbance is present (Table 2-1). The lower motor neurons are the nerve cells that transmit messages from the spinal cord to the muscle (see Figure 1-1, page 4).

TABLE 2-1

Signs and Symptoms of Lower Motor Neuron Dysfunction

Weakness
Cramps
Twitching of muscles
Muscle atrophy or thinning

Muscle twitching is common in ALS but can also occur in healthy individuals with no disease. Muscles may twitch when they are completely relaxed, recently exercised, or when there is considerable anxiety, stress, or fatigue. Twitches of muscles, in and of themselves, are not sufficient grounds for a diagnosis of ALS. Strength testing is carried out routinely in the major muscles of the limbs. The presence of weakness is common in ALS. In fact, the diagnosis of ALS cannot be made in the absence of weakness, stiffness, or clumsiness. Frequently, the weakness may be very different on one side of the body compared with the other, and occasionally it is present in only one limb. The limbs are also passively moved by the examiner to check for stiffness, a sign of the spasticity common in people with ALS. In addition to stiffness or spasticity, there may be awkwardness and slowness of movement in the hands and feet. These abnormalities reflect a disturbance in *upper motor neurons* (Table 2-2); these are the nerve cells that carry signals from the brain surface to lower motor neurons in the spinal cord (see Figure 1-1, page 4). The concept of lower and upper motor neuron disturbances is somewhat complex but is explained in detail in Chapter 1. We use these terms here because neurologists use them in coming to a diagnosis of ALS.

TABLE 2-2
Signs and Symptoms of Upper Motor Neuron Dysfunction
Incoordination
Slowing of movement
Stiffness or spasticity
Brisk reflexes
Excessive laughing or crying

The reflexes are tested with a reflex hammer. The neurologist can tell whether the reflexes are hyperactive, depressed, or absent by tapping on the knee, ankle, elbow, or wrist in specific locations. The reflexes tend to be exaggerated and very brisk in persons with ALS. Sometimes a very light tap will elicit a very strong and forceful reflex movement. Occasionally the reflexes are so active that a tap in one part of the body will elicit an excessive response in another part, a sign that supports the diagnosis of ALS. Sometimes this hyperactivity of reflexes does not appear until later in the course of the disease and, without it, the diagnosis of ALS may be difficult to make.

Tests of feeling and sensation are carried out in some detail during the examination in patients with ALS. A prominent loss of sensation would cast doubt on the diagnosis, although it does not eliminate ALS completely.

The analysis of the walking pattern is an important part of the evaluation. Patients may have difficulty rising up on their tiptoes or their heels, indicating some weakening of these muscles. They may have trouble rising from a chair without using their hands or difficulty going up or down stairs without the use of the railing. Walking may be slow and stiff, or the foot may slap or knee may buckle, all pointing to distinctive problems in nerve function.

Establishing the Diagnosis

The diagnosis of ALS depends on the presence of progressive weakness and evidence of dysfunction involving both lower and upper motor neurons. As indicated previously, lower motor neuron involvement is evidenced by muscle weakness, thinning of the muscles, twitching, cramps, and EMG abnormalities (discussed below). Lower motor neuron abnormalities are a result of degenerating motor nerve cells in the spinal cord or brainstem (the portion of the brain closest to the neck and spinal cord). Upper motor neuron abnormalities manifest as slowness, stiffness, clumsiness, awkwardness, and exaggerated reflexes. The presence of upper motor neuron abnormalities tells us that there is a degeneration of the motor nerve cells that connect the brain with the nerve cells in the spinal cord and brainstem.

Both upper motor neuron and lower motor neuron abnormalities are required for a diagnosis of ALS. A third fundamental aspect of diagnosis is a steady progression of symptoms. Symptoms that come on abruptly and then improve are not consistent with the diagnosis of ALS. Symptoms that are relieved by surgery are also inconsistent with the diagnosis of ALS. The speed of progression is highly variable in patients with ALS, but in all cases, there is a steady worsening of function.

Establishing the Diagnosis for Research Studies

Occasionally a confident diagnosis of ALS may be rendered very early in the course of the disease. The following vignette is relevant in this regard:

A 47-year-old man came for evaluation of a 2-month history of weakness and wasting in the right hand. Thinning, weakness, and twitches were present in all of the muscles of the right hand and arm, and the reflexes were abnormally active. Both his mother and his maternal uncle had died of ALS.

Comment: *The diagnosis of ALS could be made with confidence in this patient even though his symptoms were relatively short in duration because of progressive weakness, the presence of both upper motor neuron and lower motor neuron abnormalities at the time of his examination, and the positive family history. Other patients (without a family history) may have only lower motor neuron or only upper motor neuron abnormalities* *at the time of evaluation, leaving considerable difficulty in establishing a definite diagnosis except over time. The delay in diagnosis may be extremely frustrating for patients, family members, and also for the neurologist.*

The preceding discussion relates to establishing the diagnosis in a clinical and practical sense. More complex criteria have been developed for research studies in ALS, and these sometimes cause confusion for patients and families. The research criteria refer to the presence or absence of upper motor neuron and lower motor neuron signs in different regions of the body. These criteria were developed by the World Federation of Neurology and establish a level of clinical certainty of the diagnosis for research studies, depending on the evidence. They require upper and lower motor neuron abnormalities in the following four regions of the central nervous system: (1) the bulbar region, in which the speech and swallowing nerves and muscles are located; (2) the cervical region, which contains the nerves and muscles that control the arm and hands; (3) the thoracic region, which includes the muscles that control breathing and some of the abdominal muscles; and (4) the lumbosacral region, in which the leg muscles and nerves are located. There are varying degrees of certainty of diagnosis depending on the degree of involvement.

Most patients have symptoms and signs of abnormal function in only one or two regions when they are first evaluated, so a definite diagnosis of ALS by these strict criteria (which requires that three out of four areas be involved) is rarely possible until more advanced stages of the disease. Although they are useful in research, these complex standards are difficult to use in clinical practice because patients and doctors need to come to a working diagnosis that has some level of certainty.

Conditions That Can Mimic ALS

The diagnosis rarely turns out to be incorrect for the vast majority of patients diagnosed with ALS by a neurologist with expertise in ALS. Nonetheless, the following list of conditions deserves consideration because rare patients with these diseases may be confused with ALS (Table 2-3).

TABLE 2-3

Conditions That Can Mimic ALS

Cervical spine disease—pinching of the nerves of the spinal cord
Spinal muscular atrophy, Kennedy's disease (gene abnormalities causing cell degeneration)
Radiation damage
Syringomyelia (fluid sac in the spinal cord)
Hyperthyroidism and hyperparathyroidism (increased activity of the thyroid and parathyroid
   glands)
Multifocal motor neuropathies or chronic inflammatory neuropathies (inflammation of the motor
   nerves)
Lead or mercury intoxication
Lymphoma, Hodgkin's disease (forms of cancer)
Hexosaminidase deficiency (an enzyme important in nerve cell metabolism)
Post-polio syndrome (weakening that can occur 25 to 40 years after the original polio attack)
Lyme disease (caused by a bite from an infected tick)
Syphilis
HIV-AIDS

Other motor neuron diseases that may mimic ALS and may be inherited include spinal muscular atrophy as well as spinobulbar muscular atrophy (Kennedy's syndrome). Both of these diseases are very slow and gradual in their development, and they tend to be quite symmetrical, without the striking difference from one side of the body to the other side that is often seen in ALS. Kennedy's syndrome preferentially affects men and may affect the speech and swallowing muscles, as well as the limb muscles; there may be prominent twitching and thinning of the muscles, all similar to ALS. There are no upper motor neuron abnormalities in Kennedy's syndrome; other abnormalities are present including excessive breast tissue, small testicles, and numb or tingling feet. Spinal muscular atrophy is a very gradually evolving weakness of the limbs that mainly involves the lower motor neurons. Weakness and thinning in a symmetrical pattern may start at any age in both men and women.

Perhaps the most common condition that can mimic ALS is arthritis in the spine, either within the neck (*cervical region*) or in the low back (*lumbar region*). Pinching of nerves or the spinal cord may produce signs and symptoms that can be confused with ALS. Patients with disease of the spine may have lower motor neuron abnormalities, which may or may not be painful, accompanied by disturbed sensory function. Disturbance of bladder and bowel control (uncommon in ALS) and upper motor neuron signs in the legs are common in people with compression of the spinal cord from cervical spine disease. Magnetic resonance imaging (MRI) of the spine is the easiest way to evaluate the possibility of cervical or lumbar spine disease. The spinal cord may also be abnormal when there is a collection of fluid called a *syrinx* compressing the nerves. This rare abnormality is easily visualized on MRI. Any history of radiation directed toward the nerves or spinal cord that can cause degeneration in the motor neurons and the spinal cord should be carefully considered in terms of a cause of the patient's symptoms and signs.

Hormonal disorders, particularly those affecting the thyroid gland, may cause symptoms and signs that can be confused with ALS. When the thyroid gland is overactive, muscles may become thinned and weakened. All patients suspected with ALS should have thyroid function testing. Parathyroid abnormalities are rare, but they may also cause both lower motor neuron and upper motor neuron disturbances, although most patients have bone pain, numb feet, and trouble with thinking.

Patients with late onset multiple sclerosis that comes on very gradually and very slowly may also be confused with ALS. Imaging (MRI) and spinal fluid analysis and evoked response tests can usually clarify the situation.

Disorders of the immune system may cause abnormalities in the nerves that can mimic ALS. A very slowly progressive neuritis called *multifocal motor neuropathy*, caused by inflammation in the nerves, may occasionally be confused with ALS. This condition evolves extremely slowly in most patients over many years and it is rarely confused with ALS by experts. It is potentially treatable with intravenous immunoglobulin infusions. Occasionally, patients with another disorder caused by inflammation in the nerve cells called *chronic inflammatory polyneuropathy* may have so little in the way of sensory symptoms that they may be confused with ALS. This treatable condition is never associated with upper motor neuron signs, and electrodiagnostic studies document marked slowing of nerve impulses virtually never seen in ALS.

Occasionally, patients may have a toxic exposure that can mimic ALS, but this is indeed rare. Patients with lead intoxication who may develop weakness in the hands and feet are extremely rare, but this should be tested if there is a history of excessive lead exposure. The same is true of mercury intoxication, which is a very rare cause of confusion in patients suspected of ALS.

Some types of malignancy, such as leukemia, Hodgkin's disease, and lymphoma, are occasionally seen in patients with true ALS. Most of these patients have both upper motor neuron and lower motor neuron abnormalities, and the tumors may either be identified before or after ALS symptoms develop. In a very small percentage of patients, therapies to treat the tumor may help the ALS. There is a need for much more research in this particular area.

Analysis of an enzyme called *hexosaminidase A* (important in nerve cell metabolism) should be considered in patients who develop an ALS-like syndrome below the age of 30, because a deficiency of this enzyme may cause a condition mimicking ALS.

Patients who have had polio may develop a syndrome of increasing weakness 20 to 40 years after the original disease. Occasionally these patients develop ALS, perhaps unrelated to their prior polio, but most only have a modest worsening of the prior symptoms of polio. There is no specific treatment for this condition at this time.

Occasionally a muscle disease called *inclusion body myositis* may be mistaken for ALS. This is a common inflammatory muscle disease of older adults that causes weakness and muscle thinning. An electromyogram (EMG), which tests the electrical activity of muscles, may be sufficient to distinguish this muscle disease from the muscle abnormalities seen in ALS. A muscle biopsy is needed when there is a clinical suspicion of a muscle disease.

Infectious diseases rarely can mimic ALS. There has been substantial concern about Lyme disease, but thus far, few if any documented cases of Lyme disease have truly mimicked ALS.

What Tests Should Be Done?

No single test is definitive for diagnosing ALS. Most patients should have imaging studies of the brain and spinal cord (MRI), electrodiagnostic studies (EMG and nerve conduction studies), and a number of blood tests. The selection of these tests should be guided by the symptoms and abnormalities that are found during examination.

No single test is definitive for diagnosing ALS.

Imaging Study

An imaging study of the neck and cervical spine should be done when the symptoms are primarily located in the arm and hand. An MRI of the lumbar spine is indicated when there are symptoms and lower motor neuron signs that primarily involve the leg. A brain MRI will usually be needed for symptoms affecting the speech and swallowing muscles.

Electrodiagnostic Studies

The needle EMG study can help to establish the presence of nerve dysfunction in areas that are not yet symptomatic. This test can be uncomfortable. A small needle is placed in a number of muscles to record the electrical activity of the muscles. The second part of the test involves giving small electrical shocks to evaluate the speed of nerve conduction to the muscles. A primary nerve problem other than ALS is suggested if the impulse travels at slow velocities. Occasionally, such nerve problems are treatable.

Blood Tests

Blood tests should be done to evaluate blood counts and general bodily functions, including bone marrow, liver, kidney, thyroid, and parathyroid (Table 2-4). They are also used to check for inflammation of the coating of the nerve, which may be a cause of weakness in patients whose symptoms have been very long-standing. The hexosaminidase A blood test is indicated in patients under the age of 30 who have an ALS-like condition. A special DNA test is available for Kennedy's disease and this is indicated when patients have a very gradual onset of symptoms, sensory disturbances, and enlarged breast tissue. Tests for syphilis and Lyme disease—two chronic infectious diseases that in extremely rare conditions can mimic ALS—are readily available also. People with exposure to Lyme disease who have positive blood tests should possibly consider treatment under the coordination of an infectious disease specialist. In our experience, most patients who have positive Lyme tests do not improve in terms of their ALS even after extensive treatment for Lyme disease.

TABLE 2-4

Blood Tests for Diseases That Can Mimic ALS

Complete blood count:	Bone marrow disease
Chemistry panel:	Liver, kidney, thyroid disease
Intact parathormone,	
Ionized calcium:	Hyperparathyroidism
Hexosaminidase A:	ALS under age 30
Anti-GM$_1$ antibody:	Multifocal motor neuropathy
DNA analysis:	Kennedy's, spinal muscular atrophy
Lyme serology:	Tick bite, Lyme disease
MHATP:	Neurosyphilis
HIV Test:	ALS-like illness, especially with risk factors
Blood lead, mercury:	Especially with history of toxic exposure

Some people with AIDS (infection with HIV) have developed symptoms of ALS. These patients have been young, their disease has been rapidly progressive, and their spinal fluid has contained many white blood cells—usually seen in AIDS but not in ALS. Some of these individuals improved with intensive AIDS therapy and then relapsed when the viral titers rose again. Clinical trials of AIDS therapies have been negative thus far, and most experts agree that HIV infection appears unrelated to the disease process in most people with ALS.

Lower motor neuron disturbances may result from intensive long-term exposure to lead, especially in an occupational setting. Lead levels in the blood will be elevated if there is continuing lead exposure, but if such exposure is in the past, fingernail clippings and hair samples may be needed, or even a bone biopsy. Mercury intoxication is most unlikely to mimic ALS, but a blood mercury test is readily available.

The gene test for superoxide dismutase 1 (SOD-1) is commercially available, but experts agree that this test is not helpful except in families in which the disease has been present through several generations. Even in that situation, only 20 percent of families will have positive testing for

SOD-1. Fewer than 2 percent of all patients with ALS will have a positive SOD-1 test. Because of this low level of response, the SOD-1 DNA analysis is not recommended as a diagnostic test.

Muscle Biopsy

A muscle biopsy is usually only indicated in patients in whom clinical features and EMG studies raise the possibility of primary muscle disease rather than nerve disease.

Lumbar Puncture

A spinal tap to analyze spinal fluid is rarely indicated when symptoms have been present for more than 6 months. However, a spinal fluid analysis may be warranted when there is evidence of a generalized systemic disease, suspicion of multiple sclerosis, infection, or malignancy.

Receiving the News

It is extremely difficult to hear bad news, particularly when it is clear that your life will be dramatically changed compared to prior expectations. You may have a great deal of difficulty absorbing all that you are told when the diagnosis of ALS is given. Tape recording the session with the permission of the physician may be useful and allows reviewing the material later. We also recommend that you bring supportive family members and friends to the session. This is not a diagnosis to be given over the telephone, and it is much better to resist the temptation to ask for preliminary information by phone. Wait for a face-to-face discussion when you have proper support. The anxiety of anticipation and waiting for the session is understandably high, but the value of waiting until all of the testing information is available and a full discussion can be conducted in person is greatly preferred over the unsatisfactory situation of a telephone discussion. It is important to know how long it will take for lab results to return and to schedule a follow-up appointment accordingly. Obviously, an experienced expert clinician whom you trust should be the one to discuss the diagnosis rather than a person with lesser experience with whom you have no rapport.

During such a discussion, it is important to give your doctor some idea of what you already know and also what you are most worried about. This will help the doctor focus the discussion in a way that will be the most appropriate and useful for you and your family. Most people prefer a completely frank and honest discussion about the diagnosis and also what lies ahead. If you do not wish to have this kind of information, then you must make that very clear at the outset of the discussion. Each person is different in his or her preferences, and some cultural and ethnic differences will be important and should be expressed. If you and/or your family do not wish that you be given full information about the diagnosis, and would prefer that only the family be informed, this must be clearly expressed to the physician. Although this position is very unusual in large ALS centers in North America, it does occasionally occur that family members and patients prefer that the news be given to the family rather than the patient, and generally this should be honored.

In the vast majority of people, ALS is steadily progressive with a gradual and continuous loss of strength and function over time. The speed with which the disease progresses is different for every individual, and sometimes there are encouraging trends that provide hope. Fortunately, the changes in ALS occur in a gradual fashion rather than suddenly and, when difficulties arise with breathing, swallowing, or walking, there is usually plenty of advance notice and time to intervene with therapeutic support.

Preserving Hope

It is important for an individual facing ALS to look for hopeful aspects. It is almost always possible to identify a health care provider and team with expertise in caring for people who have the disease and who will commit

> It is important for an individual facing ALS to look for hopeful aspects.

to providing high quality care throughout the entire course of the disease. Developing a relationship with a multidisciplinary team of health professionals is not only reassuring and supportive, but it also provides a basis for obtaining optimal care in managing the disease.

Even though the majority of patients will survive for only 3 to 5 years beyond diagnosis, 20 percent will live beyond 5 years, and 10 percent beyond 10 years. All of us who see many patients with ALS have experience with significant numbers of patients who survive for extended periods and who preserve quality of life over many years. Factors that correlate with long-term survival are good breathing and swallowing functions; a long period of time between symptom onset and diagnosis; younger age at the time of diagnosis; the onset of symptoms in the limbs, rather than speech, swallowing, or breathing muscles; a supportive network of family and friends; a positive attitude; and a strong spiritual base. Recent studies have confirmed that survival may be extended for years by the decision to use certain interventions to prevent weight loss and swallowing and breathing difficulties. It is important to realize that, for most patients, there will be no impairment of internal organs, reasoning, or memory function. Moreover, although most people go through a period of anxiety and depression during the time of diagnosis, the vast majority emerge from the transition by adapting to the diagnosis with renewed commitment to maintaining a satisfactory quality of life. Often, antidepressant medication can speed this transition. It is critical to realize that life goes on and that many people have extraordinary quality in their lives after they adjust to the diagnosis of ALS.

There is hope in the rapidly increasing momentum of research in ALS. The number of new scientists and laboratories studying the disease, and the pace of information and discovery about the disease, has escalated rapidly in the last decade. Stem cells, gene therapy, and promising new medication in clinical trials all appear to hold tremendous promise for effective therapy in the not too distant future. Most experts agree that participation in a clinical trial is beneficial for the vast majority of patients with ALS. Participating in a clinical trial provides hope and allows for making a meaningful contribution in the battle against this disease, helping others, and possibly being helped by participation in the study. We now have one drug, riluzole (Rilutek®), which slows the progression of ALS, particularly if it is given early in the course of the disease. The drug was initially tested in patients with relatively severe, advanced ALS, and only a few months of prolonged life was observed. Subsequent studies in which the drug was started much earlier have shown more substantial benefit. The drug is safe and well tolerated, although expensive. The search is underway to find other drugs that, in combination with Rilutek®, will really put the brakes on ALS.

Why Me?

Most people cannot understand why they have developed ALS. They relentlessly search for some meaning or understanding of this turn of events. In reality, no one knows why people get this disease, except for the small percentage of patients in whom it occurs through generations of cer-

> No one knows why people get this disease.

tain families because of a genetic mutation. In the majority of patients who do not have a positive family history, we still do not know why some people get ALS and others do not. We suspect that some genes may make a person susceptible to the disease, but this has not yet been proven. We suspect that there are certain factors in the environment that may be toxic. We still do not know why certain people get this disease in spite of a rapid expansion of our understanding of the basic biology of ALS. There is a tendency to assume that something was done inappropriately or incorrectly that led to the development of ALS, or that it is a punishment for some wrongdoing. There is no evidence to support this line of thinking and it is harmful. The inspiring example of Lou Gehrig and the story of Morrie in Mitch Albom's best selling book *Tuesdays with Morrie* are about people who never really understand why they suddenly took such a difficult turn in the road of life but faced it with tremendous courage and even joy.

CHAPTER 3

Clinical Trials and Finding New Drugs for ALS

A t the present time, there is no effective medicine available to stop the progression of ALS, and no treatment available to reverse the weakness caused by this disease. Nonetheless, rapid progress in our understanding of important factors that may cause ALS is underway. A large number of clin-

> At the present time, there is no effective medicine available to stop the progression of ALS.

ical trials have already been carried out, including more than 17 major controlled trials in the last 10 years involving more than 5,000 patients. The scientific reasoning behind most of these clinical trials was discussed in Chapter 1 and is reviewed in brief below; however, a number of issues need to be addressed before discussing the individual trials.

Why Are Large Clinical Trials Necessary?

Large clinical trials are unnecessary when a new treatment has a clear-cut and dramatic beneficial effect. For example, penicillin treatment for pneumonia is dramatically effective; the fever, cough, and all symptoms begin to dramatically improve within 48 to 72 hours. Such a medication does not require a large clinical trial using a *placebo* (an inactive substance or sugar pill) to determine its effectiveness. Unfortunately, there is no treatment that will make patients dramatically better and reverse the course of ALS. In fact, we do not even have a treatment that will stop the disease from getting worse. Thus, we are in the position of testing drugs that slow down the disease progress. Unfortunately, these important effects are relatively modest and difficult to see except in a large clinical trial in which a group of patients taking the drug being studied is compared with a group of patients taking placebo.

Even though the effects of these drugs may be modest and somewhat hard to see, they may still be very significant. In both AIDS and leukemia, the first drugs studied had only a modest benefit, but by combining two or more such drugs into a combination of treatments, known as a *drug cocktail*, truly effective treatment became available for these diseases. We are pursuing the same path for ALS.

Why Participate in Clinical Trials?

Participation in clinical trials is completely voluntary. Patients are free to decline participation in a clinical trial or withdraw at any time. There are a number of very good reasons, however, why an increasing number of

> Participation in clinical trials is completely voluntary.

patients do find it gratifying to participate in clinical trials. First, participation in a clinical trial engenders the hope that springs from a very real possibility that a new drug may help you. Many people like to feel that they are making a contribution to help move the field of knowledge forward and help other people. Health care for people participating in clinical trials usually improves because of the attention that will be given to you during the regular visits that are part of every clinical trial. There is generally no cost whatsoever for participating in a clinical trial because the costs are borne by the sponsors.

However, there are risks in participating in a clinical trial. The first risk is that there may be side effects from the treatment. These are spelled out in great detail in the consent form that must be signed prior to beginning any research trial. Participants are very carefully monitored during clinical trials for the development of any serious side effects. Before a person can even be offered the chance to participate in a clinical trial, the investigators will have convinced the human research experimentation committee at their institution that the benefit outweighs the risks. Nonetheless, the decision to participate is completely voluntary. There is also a risk that participants may not receive the active drug but rather a placebo. Many people begin to have second thoughts about participating in a clinical trial when they hear that they may receive a placebo. Fortunately, many of them look at the cup as being half full rather than half empty, because *not* participating in a clinical trial brings no possibilities and no hope. Participation brings the possibility of active treatment and active involvement in the battle against ALS. Perhaps the greatest risk involved in any clinical trial for ALS is the risk of disappointment if you are part of an unsuccessful trial. This is a risk that is borne by patients and investigators together, and one which is becoming less likely as the scientific testing before a drug comes to clinical trial becomes increasingly sophisticated.

Experimental Models of ALS

When the first gene for ALS was discovered in 1993, it was finally possible to develop a good animal model to study ALS. The superoxide dismutase (SOD-1) mouse model is probably the most important breakthrough to date in our understanding of ALS. Over 100 different mutations have been found in people who have the ALS gene abnormality for SOD-1 since this initial discovery. The introduction of a gene mutation in an animal corresponds closely to the way that particular gene behaves in people with ALS. Certain gene types are correlated with very slow disease progression in patients with familial ALS, while other gene types correlate with rapid progression; these hold up in the animal model as well. Our understanding of ALS has been expanded through study of this genetic disease model. New and emerging studies using these animal models suggest the great importance of the build-up of reactive oxygen species, or *free radicals*, in the motor nerve cells. The accumulation of these oxidated substances in the motor nerves sets the stage for the development of oxidative stress, an unhealthy state for the cell. Other studies show that the energy factory of the nerve cell, the *mitochondria*, is abnormal in the mouse model and may lead to new therapeutic targets for ALS. Protein metabolism in the nerve cell is also abnormal in the mouse model and leads to the build-up of clumps of protein that interfere with nerve cell function. These and many other insights are helping us to better understand ALS and the way it develops.

Moreover, the mouse model has been tested to screen promising new agents that might be useful in treating patients with ALS. More than 100 clinical trials have been carried out with mice to screen potential new therapies. Unfortunately, the results in the animal model have not always predicted human results. Three drugs that block the effects of too much glutamate have been tested: riluzole, gabapentin, and topiramate. Riluzole (Rilutek®) did show a modest benefit on survival in both the SOD-1 mice and also in patients, a relatively close correlation for this particular drug. Gabapentin (Neurontin®) showed a modest benefit in mice, but none could be demonstrated in two large clinical trials in patients with ALS. A number of drugs, such as topiramate (Topamax®), have shown no effect on mice and also no benefit in patients. Several trials are underway currently, because of promising results in the mouse model, in the hope that this will also be proven to be beneficial in patients, including coenzyme Q-10, celecoxib (Celebrex®), and minocycline (Minocin®). These drugs support mitochondrial function (coenzyme Q-10), reduce inflammation (celecoxib and minocycline), or block preprogrammed cell death (minocycline).

Recently a rat model was developed with the SOD-1 mutation that will make it easier to do more comprehensive studies on this larger animal. Three new genes (alsin, dynactin, and senataxin) have been discovered recently that may lead to important new mouse models that will undoubtedly expand our understanding of the disease process and may prove more useful in screening new drugs.

Clinical trials in ALS have substantially improved over the years. This was greatly enhanced by the publication of *Guidelines for the Conduct of Clinical Trials in ALS* (see Table 3-1). The next section is an overview of the new guidelines and is given in the spirit of helping patients understand some of the issues that are addressed to ensure the very best quality of ALS clinical trials.

Guidelines for Clinical Trials

In April 1994, a group of ALS specialists from countries all over the world met for 3 days to develop guidelines for clinical trials. These guidelines were revised in April 1998 (Table 3-1). The newer guidelines were designed to improve the efficiency of trial design; increase the consistency of data analysis; include patients in clinical trials who are at an earlier stage in the disease process; adopt the new CONSORT (Consolidated Standards of Reports and Trials) Guidelines that will make comparisons among studies easier; protect the interests of patients who enroll in a clinical trial; define quality of life measures; and propose better methods for collaboration between industry and investigators.

In 1997, many major neurology and internal medicine journals adopted the CONSORT Guidelines and established them as mandatory reporting criteria for all clinical trials. It is clear from a review of earlier trials that poor methodology and poor reporting often yielded biased results. A checklist of twenty-one items in the CONSORT Guidelines must be taken into account in advance during the design phase and must be adhered to during the reporting process for all clinical trials. This new standard has raised the quality of all clinical trials.

It is difficult to reconcile some differences in clinical trials. The diagnosis must be firm, but it is highly desirable to include patients in the very early stages of the disease. Large-scale trials are more likely to provide a conclusive result, but small screening trials are much more cost-effective. Unfortunately, quick small trials often are inconclusive. Small inconclusive trials sometimes fail to detect the beneficial effect of a drug that may have a modest effect (false negative results), whereas a larger more expensive trial may have shown the drug to be beneficial. On the other hand, small trials sometimes give misleading (false positive) results, leading people to believe that a drug may be helpful in treating a disease when really it has no value at all. This false positive effect appears to have occurred in the first multicenter gabapentin (Neurontin®) trial.

TABLE 3-1
Consensus Guidelines for ALS Clinical Trials

Diagnosis

1. The diagnosis in accordance with the World Federation of Neurology, El Escorial Criteria.

Inclusion

2. Both sporadic and familial ALS can be entered into most trials.
3. Entry should be limited to patients between the ages of 18 and 85.
4. Before entry there should be evidence of progression during a period of 6 months from onset of symptoms but not more than 5 years.

Exclusion

5. Patients with significant sensory abnormalities, dementia, other neurologic diseases, uncompensated medical illness, substance abuse, and psychiatric illness should be excluded. The patient should not be taking other investigational drugs.

Endpoints

6. Primary and secondary endpoints should be defined in advance; muscle strength and death or ventilator dependence are at present the most useful primary endpoints for a therapeutic trial.

Controls

7. All trials should include a control group.

Quality-of-Life

8. An ALS-specific quality-of-life assessment should be developed and incorporated into every efficacy trial.

Statistical Analyses

9. Trials should be designed with à priori defined statistical analysis.

"Compassionate Release" and Treatment IND

10. "Compassionate release" and treatment INDs should generally be used but therapeutic efficacy of the drug must not be compromised.

Release of Information and Investigators' Responsibility

11. The manner in which information is released during and after a trial should be defined in the protocol. It is recommended that no efficacy results be released until peer review publication is imminent, other than at scientific meetings.
12. It is the investigator's responsibility to assure that commercial concerns do not distort the conduct of the trial.

Clinical Trial Phases

13. ALS trials should be organized in three phases. Phase I trials are conducted to obtain toxicity and pharmacokinetic information. Phase II trials (pilot, exploratory, screening) are performed for dose finding, preliminary efficacy assessment, and further safety observations. Phase III studies are designed to determine definitive efficacy and safety.
14. Phase I trials should incorporate concurrent placebo control and should be continued for 6 months, depending on the design.

TABLE 3-1

Consensus Guidelines for ALS Clinical Trials (continued)

15. Phase II trials may use concurrent placebo controls, historic controls, or a crossover design. This phase is used to screen agents with potential therapeutic value. If improvement in strength or function is the endpoint, the trial should last at least 6 months. If stabilization or slowing of deterioration is the endpoint, the trial should last a minimum of 12 months, depending on the nature of the drug.
16. Phase III trials should be placebo-controlled. This trial should include analysis of time to death, assessment of strength measured by maximum voluntary isometric contraction, pulmonary function, and functional performance by the ALS rating scale.

Data and Safety Monitoring Board

17. An independent data and safety monitoring board should be established. This should consist of independent physicians and biostatisticians who periodically review all data during the conduct of the trial and at its conclusion. This committee is also responsible for safeguarding against scientific fraud. It is essential that this committee be free of conflict of interest and acting on the patients' behalf.

Abbreviation: IND = investigational new drug
Source: Modified from The World Federation of Neurology Research Group on Neuromuscular Disease Subcommittee on Motor Neuron Disease: Airlie House Guidelines. Miller RG, Munsat TL, Swash M, Brooks BR. Consensus guidelines for the design and implementation of clinical triials in ALS. J Neurol Sci 1999; 169:2–12., with kind permission from Elsevier Science – NL, Sara Burgerhartstraat 25, 1055 KV Amsterdam, The Netherlands.

Now that we have a single approved drug, riluzole (Rilutek®), most patients take riluzole while they also participate in a clinical trial. Although patients do not like the idea of placebo-controlled trials and would rather receive an active drug, the FDA and the NIH both require placebo-controlled trials to show the effectiveness of any drug in ALS. All ALS trials will include a placebo for at least the foreseeable future. Survival is certainly an important endpoint in all clinical trials, but this requires a much longer and more costly trial than those that use a functional measure of effectiveness, such as muscle strength, functional scales, or quality of life (Tables 3-2 to 3-5). Researchers must make decisions regarding cost and other considerations in every clinical trial, and the new guidelines provide some help (Table 3-1).

The updated clinical trial guidelines contain recommendations that quality of life must be measured in all clinical trials (the Short Form 36, Table 3-5). An ALS-specific quality-of-life instrument would be preferable for ALS clinical trials.

TABLE 3-2

ALS Assessment Techniques

ALS Global Scales (Clinimetric Tests)

Scores based on subjective or historic data
    ALS functional rating scale
    ALS severity scale
Scores based on clinical tests
    Norris scale
    Appel scale
Scales used for ALS and other diseases
    Schwab and England global rating scale
    Ashworth spasticity scale

Muscle Strength Testing

Quantitative tests
    Maximum voluntary isometric contraction
    Handheld dynamometer
    Manual muscle testing

Electrophysiologic Testing

Compound muscle action potentials
Motor unit number estimate

Quality-of-Life Assessment

Short form – 36 (SF-36)
Short form – 12 (SF-12)
Sickness Impact Profile

ALS clinical trials involving new unapproved drugs generally are carried out initially in small numbers of patients to obtain information about toxicity and tolerability (phase I). In most instances, patients are randomly assigned to receive active drug or placebo and safety is the main objective. Neither the patient nor the physician knows what they are assigned to receive; this situation is referred to as *double-blind*. The focus is on the safety and side effects of the drug in this type of phase I trial, and effectiveness in slowing the disease progress is not a major objective. In the screening trial (phase II), drug effectiveness is a major focus and some safety data are generally obtained as well. In most instances, these also involve both a drug and placebo group. Screening trials are generally designed to include 100 to 200 patients, and different doses and measurements may be

TABLE 3-3

ALS Functional Rating Scale—Revised*

1. Speech
    4. Normal speech processes
    3. Detectable speech disturbance
    2. Intelligible with repeating
    1. Speech combined with nonvocal communication
    0. Loss of useful speech.

The rest are all similarly graded into 4 (normal) to 0 (complete loss of function)

2. Salivation (4 to 0)
3. Swallowing (4 to 0)
4. Handwriting (4 to 0)
5a. Cutting food and handling utensils (patients without gastrostomy) (4 to 0)†
5b. Preparing tube food and handling device (patients with gastrostomy) (4 to 0)†
6. Dressing and hygiene (4 to 0)
7. Turning in bed and adjusting bedclothes (4 to 0)
8. Walking (4 to 0)
9. Climbing stairs (4 to 0)
10. Dyspnea (4 to 0)
11. Orthopnea (4 to 0)
12. Respiratory insufficiency (4 to 0)

*Point scores range from 0 (maximum impairment) to 4.0 (healthy).
†5a is used for those who take oral food and 5b is used for those who use only gastrostomy tube feeding.
Source: Adapted from the ALS CNTF Treatment Study (ACTS) Phase I-II Study Group: The amyotrophic lateral sclerosis functional rating scale: Assessment of activities of daily living in patients with amyotrophic lateral sclerosis. *Arch Neurol* 1996; 53:141–147.

examined to identify optimal trial design for a phase III trial. The conclusive phase III study usually involves large numbers of patients (often as many as 1,000 to 1,200) and may include more than one dose, again comparing drug to placebo. Phase IV studies are conducted after the drug has been licensed for marketing in order to detect safety concerns that may occur as the drug is used in larger numbers of patients. The inclusion and exclusion criteria vary for each study, but representative criteria for many studies are described in Table 3-1.

Other issues in trial design include the importance of randomization to minimize prejudice toward a certain result—either positive or negative. In the randomizing process, a patient is assigned by chance to either receive active drug or placebo in a double-blind fashion, such that neither patient

TABLE 3-4

Appel Scale

1. Bulbar (6–30)
   Swallowing (3–15)
   Speech (3–15)
2. Respiratory—FVC (6–30)
3. Muscle strength—MMT by MRC scales (6–36)
   Upper extremities (sum of R and L sides) (2–14)
   Lower extremities (sum of R and L sides) (2–14)
   Grip (pounds R grip plus L grip divided by 2) (1–4)
   Lateral pinch (pounds R pinch plus L pinch divided by 2) (1–4)
4. Muscle function—lower extremities (6–35)
   Standing from chair in seconds (1–5)
   Standing from lying supine in seconds (1–6)
   Walking 20 ft (6 m) (1–5)
   Need for assistive devices (1–5)
   Climbing and descending four standard steps in seconds (1–6)
   Hips and legs (behavioral) (1–8)
5. Muscle function—upper extremities (6–33)
   Dressing and feeding (behavioral) (1–4)
   Propelling wheelchair 20 ft (6 m) in seconds (1–6)
   Arms and shoulders (grades the most affected side) (1–6)
   Cutting theraplast—dominant hand in seconds (1–6)
   Purdue pegboard (60s)—number of pegs R side plus number of pegs L side divided by 2 (1–5)
   Block (60s)—number of blocks R side plus number of blocks L side divided by 2 (1–5)

* Point scores range from 30 (healthy) to 164 (maximum impairment), derived by totaling scores from all test items (score ranges in parentheses).
Abbreviations: FVC = forced vital capacity, MMT = manual muscle testing, MRC = Medical Research Council.
Source: Adapted from Appel V, et al. A rating scale for amyotrophic lateral sclerosis: description and preliminary experience. *Ann Neurol* 1987;22:328-333.

nor evaluator knows what the patient is taking. As noted above, under these circumstances, the trial is much more likely to give a reliable result.

A number of safeguards for protecting patients in clinical trials have been developed. Patients must be fully informed not only about their par-

Patients must be fully informed not only about their participation in the trial, but about their diagnosis and what they can expect in the future.

TABLE 3-5

Short Form–36 (SF-36 HEALTH SURVEY)

INSTRUCTIONS: This questionnaire asks for your views about your health. This information will help keep track of how you feel and how well you are able to perform your usual activities.

Please answer every question by marking one box. If you are unsure about how to answer, please give the best answer that you can.

I. In general, would you say your health is:

☐	☐	☐	☐	☐
Excellent	Very good	Good	Fair	Poor

II. *Compared to one year ago,* how would you rate your health in general now? (Check one box)
- ☐ Much better now than one year ago
- ☐ Somewhat better now than one year ago
- ☐ About the same as one year ago
- ☐ Somewhat worse now than one year ago
- ☐ Much worse now than one year ago

III. The following items are about activities you might do during a typical day. Does *your health now limit you* in these activities? If so, how much?

	Yes, Limited A lot	Yes, Limited A Little	No, Not Limited At All
1. **Vigorous activities**, such as running, lifting heavy objects, participating in strenuous sports	☐	☐	☐
2. **Moderate activities**, such as moving a table, pushing a vacuum cleaner, bowling, or playing golf	☐	☐	☐
3. Lifting or carrying groceries	☐	☐	☐
4. Climbing several flights of stairs	☐	☐	☐
5. Climbing one flight of stairs	☐	☐	☐
6. Bending, kneeling, or stooping	☐	☐	☐
7. Walking more than a kilometer or 2/3 of a mile	☐	☐	☐
8. Walking several blocks	☐	☐	☐
9. Walking one block	☐	☐	☐
10. Bathing or dressing yourself	☐	☐	☐

IV. During the *past 4 weeks,* have you had any of the following problems with your work or other regular daily activities *as a result of your physical health?*

	YES	NO
1. Cut down on the **amount of time** you spent on work or other activities	☐	☐
2. **Accomplished less** than you would like	☐	☐
3. Were limited in the **kind** of work or other activities	☐	☐
4. Had difficulty performing the work or other activities (for example, it took extra effort)	☐	☐

TABLE 3-5
Short Form–36 (SF-36 HEALTH SURVEY)

V. During *the past 4 weeks*, have you had any of the following problems with your work or other regular daily activities *as a result of any emotional problems* (such as feeling depressed or anxious)?

	YES	NO
1. Cut down the **amount of time** you spend on work or other activities	☐	☐
2. **Accomplished less** than you would like	☐	☐
3. Didn't do work or other activities as carefully as usual	☐	☐

VI. During the *past 4 weeks*, to what extent has your physical health or emotional problems interfered with your *normal social activities* with family, friends, neighbors, or groups? (Check the box that applies.)

☐ Not at all ☐ Quite a bit
☐ Slightly ☐ Extremely
☐ Moderately

VII. How much *bodily pain* have you had during the *past 4 weeks* (check the box which applies)?

☐ None ☐ Moderate
☐ Very mild ☐ Severe
☐ Mild ☐ Very severe

VIII. During the *past 4 weeks*, how much did *pain* interfere with your normal work (including both work outside the home and housework)? (Check the box that applies.)

☐ Not at all ☐ Quite a bit
☐ Very mild ☐ Extremely
☐ Mild

IX. These questions are about how you feel and how things have been with you *during the past 4 weeks*. For each question, please give the one answer that comes closest to the way you have been feeling. How much of the time during the *past 4 weeks*:

	All of the Time	Most of the Time	A Good Bit of the Time	Some of the Time	A Little of the Time	None of the Time
1. Did you feel full of pep?	☐	☐	☐	☐	☐	☐
2. Have you been a very nervous person?	☐	☐	☐	☐	☐	☐
3. Have you felt so down in the dumps that nothing could cheer you up?	☐	☐	☐	☐	☐	☐
4. Have you felt calm and peaceful?	☐	☐	☐	☐	☐	☐
5. Did you have a lot of energy?	☐	☐	☐	☐	☐	☐
6. Have you felt downhearted and blue?	☐	☐	☐	☐	☐	☐

		All of the Time	Most of the Time	A Good Bit of the Time	Some of the Time	A Little of the Time	None of the Time
7.	Did you feel worn out?	☐	☐	☐	☐	☐	☐
8.	Have you been a happy person?	☐	☐	☐	☐	☐	☐
9.	Did you feel tired?	☐	☐	☐	☐	☐	☐

X. During the *past 4 weeks*, how much of the time has your *physical health or emotional problems* interfered with your social activities (like visiting with friends, relatives, etc.)?

All of the Time	Most of the Time	Some of the Time	A Little of the Time	None of the Time
☐	☐	☐	☐	☐

XI. How TRUE or FALSE is each of the following statements for you?
(Check the box that applies on each line.)

		Definitely True	Mostly True	Don't Know	Mostly False	Definitely False
1.	I seem to get sick a little easier than other people.	☐	☐	☐	☐	☐
2.	I am as healthy as anybody I know.	☐	☐	☐	☐	☐
3.	I expect my health to get worse.	☐	☐	☐	☐	☐
4.	My health is excellent.	☐	☐	☐	☐	☐

Source: Ware JE, Jr., Sherbourne CD: The MOS 36-Item Short-form Health Survey (SF-36). I. Conceptional framework and item selection, *Medical Care* 1992;30:473-83.

ticipation in the trial, but about their diagnosis and wht they can expect in the future (Table 3-6). Trials must be designed to minimize the psychological and physical burden on patients, and discrimination must be strictly avoided in screening patients for trials.

An Independent Safety Monitoring Committee is selected in advance of every clinical trial. There should be a balance between expert ALS clinicians and statisticians and representatives from industry (in pharmaceutical-sponsored trials), with a majority of academic people on the committee. It is also desirable to have a patient advocate on the Steering Committee. This structure provides a fair balance to ensure that test standards are met.

The ways in which results will be made public should also be agreed upon in advance. The results should be released in a peer-reviewed scientific meeting, but they should be shared with investigators from each site and with participating patients before they are released to the media. Timely publication of the results is important as well.

TABLE 3-6
Key Elements of Informed Consent

Statement of purpose
- Explain procedures
- Potential risks and discomforts
- Potential benefits
- Alternative procedures
- Assurance of confidentiality
- Potential research-related injury
- Questions
- Participation is voluntary
- Participant costs

Other details regarding the clinical trial guidelines can be found on the World Federation of Neurology Web site (see Resources, page 63).

Standards of Care

Providing the very best standard of health care management is essential for all patients with ALS. There is at present no universally agreed upon stan-

> Providing the very best standard of health care management is essential for all patients with ALS.

dard to provide a background of care that is uniform for patients in clinical trials. The American Academy of Neurology recently sponsored an evidence-based process for developing a practice parameter for the management of ALS. The practice parameter was the result of a large literature review. It approaches five major issues in ALS, including breaking the news (telling the diagnosis), symptomatic therapy (beginning with saliva control and uncontrolled or excessive laughing and crying), nutrition and feeding tubes (*percutaneous endoscopic gastrostomy*), management of breathing difficulty, and end-of-life care. These practice parameters should help raise the standard of care for patients with ALS and provide a more uniform basis for the care of patients in clinical trials.

What We Have Learned from Clinical Trials

The next section provides an overview of the types of therapies that have been tested in clinical trials. For each therapy, a brief explanation is provided as to the reasons for testing this class of compounds. The different designs of trials are also discussed. For some readers, this section will be used only as a pertinent reference to look up a specific agent, while others will be interested in much of the detail.

Drug Testing in Clinical Trials

Although the cause of ALS is still unknown, an *excitotoxicity* from the amino acid glutamate, which causes damage to motor neurons, may play an important role. In brief, evidence from a number of experiments suggests that an excess of glutamate can damage motor neurons and that high concentrations of glutamate are present in the blood and spinal fluid of many patients with ALS. Glutamate removal is defective in the motor areas of the brain and spinal cord in patients with ALS due to a defect in key proteins.

Riluzole (Rilutek®)

Riluzole (Rilutek®) blocks the build-up of glutamate and reduces nerve damage in a number of experimental models. It was thought that the anti-glutamate properties of riluzole might be beneficial in patients with ALS and clinical trials were begun. Preclinical data with riluzole indicated prolonged survival and also preserved function in the mutant SOD-1 mouse model of ALS. Moreover, the results of human trials indicated prolonged survival in patients taking riluzole compared with those taking placebo (Figure 3-1). These trials demonstrated a survival benefit of a few months on average for patients taking riluzole as opposed to placebo (Table 3-7). Data from large studies suggest that the benefit may be greater when the drug is given earlier in the course of the disease, thereby prolonging survival for a longer period. Quality of life was not examined directly in these studies, although some data suggest that patients who took riluzole remained in better health for a longer period of time compared to those

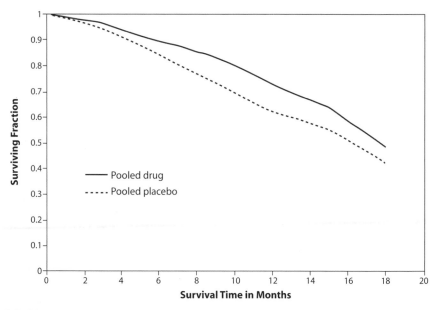

FIGURE 3-1

Actuarial survival curves for combined results from three clinical trials of riluzole. The curve at the upper right documents modestly longer survival for those taking riluzole.

Source: adapted from Miller R, et al. Riluzole for amyotrophic lateral sclerosis/motor neuron disease (*Cochrane Review*). The Cochrane Library 2004 (1): Oxford: Update Software.

patients taking placebo. Taken together, these data suggest there is an advantage to taking the drug in earlier stages of the disease as compared with the late stages.

A 57-year-old woman with ALS had progressive weakness of the legs over a period of 30 months. The diagnosis of ALS appeared secure. Her breathing, speech, and swallowing function were normal and she wanted to know whether riluzole should be taken to slow down the progression of the disease. She had been told by her local doctor that the beneficial effect is trivial and not worth the expense, but she scheduled an appointment at an ALS center for a second opinion.

Comment: *At present, riluzole is the only drug of documented benefit and the only drug approved for ALS by the Food and*

TABLE 3-7

Recent Phase III Studies in ALS

Design	Riluzole	IGF-1	Gabapentin	Xaliproden	Subcut. BDNF*
Centers	31	8	15	40	20
Patients	959	236	204	2000	350
Diagnosis	El Escorial	"ALS"	El Escorial	El Escorial	El Escorial
Exclusion	VC < 60%, > 5 yr	VC < 60% > 115 Baylor Scores > 3 yr	VC < 60%, > 3 yr, Riluzole	Two studies, one with riluzole VC < 60%, < 6 mo, > 5 yr	FVC < 60, > 90% > 5 yr ALSFRS < 18
Dose levels	3	2	1	2	1
Study period	18 mo.	9 mo.	9 mo.	18 mo.	12 mo.
Primary outcome	Death, tracheostomy, ventilator	Baylor scores	MVIC	VC/Death, tracheostomy, ventilator	Death, continuous ventilator dependence
Secondary outcomes	MRC Modified Norris FVC CGIC VAS	SIP Survival	Arm megascore Timed function FVC ALSFRS Survival Symptom survey	MRC ALSFRS VAS, Functional scales CGIC SIP	VC ALSFRS
Results	At 18 months, 50% of placebo-treated patients and 57% of those with 100 mg dose still alive	Baylor scores and SIP deteriorated less with higher dose	No differences	Results equivocal	No benefit
Problems	Insensitive measurement techniques, variability in testing	Stringent inclusion criteria, European study not robust, but supportive	Unbalanced symptom duration at baseline	Confounding effect of riluzole	Discontinuation too early?

* High dose BDNF subcutaneously. An intrathecal study is also complete.

Abbreviations: ALSFRS = ALS functional rating scale; CGIC = clinical global impression of changes; El Escorial = WFN El Escorial ALS Diagnostic Criteria; VC = vital capacity; IGF-1 = insulin-like growth factor-1; MRC = Medical Research Council; MVIC = maximum voluntary isometric contraction; SIP = sickness impact profile; VAS = visual assessment scale

Drug Administration in the United States. It has also been approved in Europe and provisionally in Canada. The drug was the subject of a practice advisory for clinicians published by the American Academy of Neurology and also by the Cochrane Collaboration, a global evidence-based medicine consortium (see Resources, page 63).

There is convincing evidence that the progression of ALS is slowed on the basis of controlled clinical trials. It is true that the therapeutic effect is not dramatic and that neither physicians nor patients can observe a therapeutic benefit from taking riluzole in any one individual. However, an analysis of the combined data from both trials demonstrated a 40 percent reduction in the risk of death at 12 months for patients taking riluzole as compared with placebo. The average prolongation of survival was approximately 3 months. Recent studies suggest that starting riluzole early in the course of the disease, or in patients with a slower than usual form of the disease, may produce greater benefit. The patient described in the vignette above has already demonstrated a slow rate of progression, and with normal swallowing and breathing function, her chances for long-term survival are very good. We would recommend riluzole for her if it is not a financial hardship and, in fact, most patients with ALS take this drug. Riluzole is expensive (approximately $835 per month in the United States), but many third-party payers cover the cost and most patients can take the drug with few, if any, side effects.

A 42-year-old man with a 6-month history of progressive weakness and wasting of the hands was recently diagnosed with ALS. He had already heard about riluzole but his doctor warned him that the risk of liver damage was so high that the drug was probably not worthwhile.

Comment: *Both the data from the placebo-controlled trials of riluzole and subsequent clinical experience with the drug indicate that safety is not a major issue with riluzole. Modestly abnormal liver function blood tests were found in some* *patients, although it is rarely necessary to discontinue the drug because of a serious elevation of liver function tests. Nonetheless, to be safe, liver function blood tests must be obtained monthly for the first 3 months and then at intervals of 3 months thereafter. In the small number of patients who develop significant elevations in liver function, the condition is usually readily reversible by tapering the dose or discontinuing the drug. Clinical experience suggests similarities between riluzole and a number of other widely used medications in which serious liver problems are extremely rare.*

Other side effects, particularly nausea, may be troubling to people who do not start at a low dose and increase the dose gradually. The recommended dose of 50 mg at 12-hour intervals on an empty stomach is difficult for most patients to tolerate in the beginning. Our procedure is to start the first dose on a full stomach after dinner for a week, add a second pill after breakfast for another week, and then, if the drug is well tolerated, to gradually increase the interval after dinner and after breakfast to the point where the drug is being taken on an empty stomach to maximize its absorption. Fatigue is common in ALS and may be increased when taking riluzole. Many patients with disturbed sleep, depression, and marked weakness requiring expenditure of greater energy to accomplish daily tasks have other reasons for fatigue besides riluzole. We frequently interrupt administration of the drug if fatigue becomes marked to assess its contribution to fatigue, which is usually quite modest.

A number of other agents have been or are being tested for possible therapeutic effectiveness in ALS, as described below. They include a number of antiepileptic drugs that have antiglutamate actions and may be effective in ALS.

Gabapentin (Neurontin®)

Gabapentin is one of the antiepileptic drugs that may have an antiglutamate action in ALS. In studies both in tissue culture and in the SOD-1 mouse model, there was prolonged survival of motor neurons and experimental animals with ALS using gabapentin. A phase II, placebo-controlled study that involved 152 patients with ALS was inconclusive but showed a trend towards a beneficial effect. Gabapentin was generally well tolerated; the most common side effects were dizziness or lightheadedness, drowsiness, and fatigue.

Encouraged by these results, a phase III placebo-controlled trial of 204 patients was undertaken (Table 3-7). This larger, longer, and higher dose study was completely negative, showing no benefit for patients taking gabapentin compared to placebo.

Branched-Chain Amino Acids

Branched-chain amino acids (leucine, isoleucine, and valine), which are widely available in health food stores, were thought to potentially interrupt the toxic effects of excess glutamate on nerve cells. Unfortunately, several clinical trials failed to find a beneficial therapeutic effect.

Dextromethorphan (Benylin®)

Dextromethorphan, a compound that blocks one type of glutamate receptor, has been evaluated in four randomized controlled trials. Unfortunately, all of the trials have demonstrated no therapeutic benefit.

Lamotrigine (Lamictal®)

Lamotrigine, an antiepileptic drug that might have a beneficial effect upon glutamate excitotoxicity, was tested only in very low doses of 100 mg/day in 67 patients in a randomized, controlled trial. The primary endpoint was survival. After 18 months, no significant differences were found between patients taking drug versus placebo, but further trials at higher doses might be warranted.

Topiramate (Topamax®)

The anticonvulsant topiramate, which appeared to be effective in some models of glutamate toxicity, was recently studied in a 1-year placebo-controlled trial involving 300 patients. This study was completely negative and no beneficial effect was found.

Calcium Channel Blockers

Calcium channel blockers have been evaluated in combination with other drugs (riluzole and creatine) that show a benefit in the mouse model of ALS. There have been two controlled clinical trials in patients. The first involved verapamil (Verelan®) in seventy-two patients and no benefit was found. Nimodipine (Nimotop®) showed promise in the mouse model and was evaluated in eight-seven patients during 3 months of treatment compared to 3 months of placebo; no benefit was found in these brief studies.

Nerve Growth Factors

Neurotrophic factors are substances that can nourish and prolong survival of motor nerve cells in laboratory-based experiments. This class of therapeutic agents was thought initially to have substantial promise for ALS. Unfortunately, thus far, the promise has yet to be fulfilled in human trials.

Thyrotrophin Releasing Hormone (TRH)

TRH was the first neurotrophic factor to raise a good deal of interest as a potential treatment for patients with ALS in the early 1980s. Four open-label (no placebo) trials of TRH were reported with mixed results. Subsequently, it took five controlled trials, all showing no benefit, to convince the ALS community that this compound was of no value as a treatment for ALS.

The Injectable, Insulin-Like Growth Factor 1 (Myotrophin)

Myotrophin has been studied in two trials, one in the United States and one in Europe. The study in the United States demonstrated a beneficial effect (Table 3-7), with high-dose patients experiencing greater slowing of loss of function compared with low dose and placebo (Figure 3-2). In addition, this

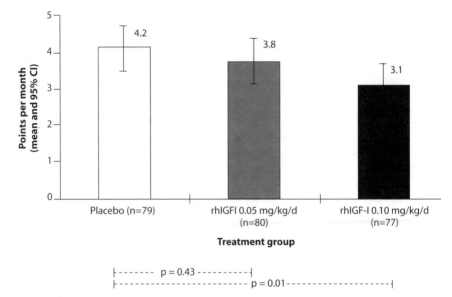

FIGURE 3-2

Rate of disease symptom progression of the three treatment groups expressed as average change in points per month (Appel ALS Rating Scale total score slope) (n=236 patients). The high-dose group experienced a 1.1 point per month or 26 percent slower rate of symptom progression when compared with the placebo group (p = 0.01). A dose-response relationship was observed. rhIGF-1 = recombinant human insulin-like growth factor-1.

Source: Adapted from Lai EC, et al. Effect of recombinant human insulin-like growth factor-I on progression of ALS. A placebo-controlled study. The North America ALS/IGF-I Study Group. *Neurology* 1997; 49:1621-1630.

was the first trial of any agent in ALS in which a slowing of the loss of quality of life was demonstrated (Figure 3-3). Again, there was a greater maintenance of quality of life in the high-dose group, modest maintenance in the low-dose group, and none with placebo. Unfortunately, a smaller European study did not show positive results. A third study is currently underway with funding from the NIH to settle the question of whether this agent is beneficial to patients with ALS.

Ciliary Neurotrophic Factor (CNTF)

Two controlled trials of CNTF, another injectable nerve growth factor, were carried out in the United States. One trial involved 570 patients for

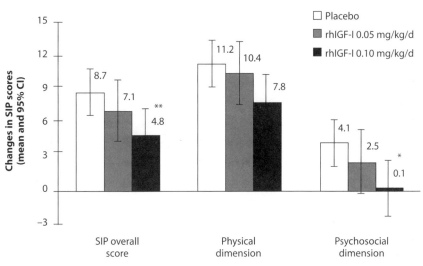

FIGURE 3-3

Changes from baseline to the last assessment in the Sickness Impact Profile (SIP) in the three treatment groups. Differences between the high-dose and placebo groups were statistically significant for the overall (p = 0.01) and psychosocial dimension (p = 0.02) scores.* p ≤ 0.05 compared with the placebo group;** p ≤ 0.01 compared with the placebo group.

Source: Adapted from Lai EC, et al. Effect of recombinant human insulin-like growth factor-I on progression of ALS. A placebo-controlled study. The North America ALS/IGF-I Study Group. *Neurology* 1997; 49:1621-1630.

6 months, and the other involved 730 patients studied over a 9-month period. No significant benefit was found in either of these large trials.

Growth Hormone (GH)

GH injections were compared with placebo for up to 18 months in a controlled trial involving seventy-five patients. Again, no significant benefit was found for patients taking growth hormone compared with placebo.

Gangliosides

Gangliosides enhance the sprouting of nerve cells and prolong their survival. Three controlled trials have been conducted involving forty patients in each trial. All showed no benefit after 3 or 6 months.

Brain-Derived Neurotrophic Factor (BDNF)

BDNF is a naturally occurring neurotrophic substance that has powerful preclinical effects on the survival of motor neurons in animal models and in cells grown in culture; however, BDNF was ineffective at changing the neurodegeneration seen in the ALS mouse model. Regeneron sponsored a large trial of BDNF injected under the skin that showed no convincing overall result. Some patients developed diarrhea, indicating a biological effect of the drug in those patients who had higher levels of BDNF in their blood. This subgroup of patients showed a beneficial response to the drug. Thus, two further studies of BDNF were carried out with (1) higher doses injected under the skin (Table 3-7), and (2) injected directly into the spinal fluid that bathes the brain and spinal cord. Both of these large trials were entirely without benefit for patients with ALS in spite of these very aggressive approaches.

Glial-Cell Derived Neurotrophic Factor (GDNF)

GDNF has been under development for ALS clinical trials. Administration of GDNF directly into the fluid that bathes the brain failed to produce clinical benefit for patients with ALS. These studies, which began in 1996, were suspended because of the lack of efficacy and the occurrence of significant side effects. Very recent encouraging results with direct injection of GDNF in the brain in Parkinson's disease patients may prompt further consideration of GDNF in ALS.

Xaliproden

Studies of another promising neurotrophic factor that can be taken orally were sponsored by Sanofi. This compound (SR57746A) appeared to slow the decline of respiratory function in a phase II trial. The phase III trial was 18 months in duration and involved approximately 2,000 patients in a placebo-controlled design (Table 3-7). The results were encouraging but inconclusive, and were not sufficient for the drug to be approved by regulatory agencies for use in ALS.

Small Molecule Neurotrophic Agents

Neuroimmunophilins are a new class of small molecules that have neurotrophic properties; they can be taken by mouth and do not need to be injected. These orally active agents represent a new approach to treatment of neurodegenerative diseases such as ALS but they are not yet available for ALS trials.

Selegeline (Deprenyl®)

This is a drug that has shown promise in slowing the progress of Parkinsonism. It was evaluated in two controlled trials involving 121 patients with ALS in a 6-month trial. No significant benefit from selegeline was found in ALS.

Antioxidants

Acetylcysteine

A controlled trial involving 111 patients over 12 months compared the antioxidant *acetylcysteine*, injected under the skin, with placebo. There was a favorable trend on survival after 1 year in patients treated with the antioxidant, but no significant differences in disease progression were observed between the two groups.

Vitamin E

A dose of 1,000 mg/day of vitamin E plus riluzole was compared with riluzole alone in a recent European study involving 289 patients with ALS who were studied for 1 year. Biochemical markers of oxidative stress, causing a build-up of toxic substances of metabolism, were measured in the blood in a subset of patients at entry and after 3 months of treatment. There was no significant difference in the primary effectiveness measure, but there was a slower progression from the milder health state to a more severe health state in patients taking vitamin E. Moreover, after 3 months of treatment, there was an improvement in blood markers of oxidative stress in patients taking vitamin E in combination with riluzole. We recommend vitamin E, 2000 i.u. per day, taken with milk in the morning.

Coenzyme Q-10

Coenzyme Q-10 is a widely available antioxidant that appeared in one study to have a beneficial effect in Parkinson's disease. High doses of this compound will be evaluated in a study coordinated by Columbia University and funded by NIH.

> *A 47-year-old man with a 4-month history of progressive painless weakness in the arms and legs was found to have ALS. At his first follow-up appointment after receiving the diagnosis, he wanted advice about alternative therapies including vitamins and antioxidants.*

> **Comment:** *Thus far there has been no evidence from clinical trials that any regimen involving antioxidants, vitamins, or other alternative therapies is effective in slowing disease progression in ALS. Vitamin E delayed the onset of motor neuron disease in an ALS mouse model. In a controlled trial in patients, vitamin E prolonged the period of time when patients were in a better state of health. There was a beneficial trend from acetylcysteine but no statistical significant benefit in one controlled trial. Creatine has not demonstrated benefit in two human trials. Every clinic director has a list of other alternative therapies, but as yet the evidence is scant about effectiveness. These alternative treatments are discussed in more detail in Chapter 6.*

Immunosuppressive Therapy

Cyclophosphamide (Cytoxan®)

Cyclophosphamide, a powerful agent that suppresses the immune system, has been evaluated in two uncontrolled trials (trials without using a placebo control) in ALS. These studies were undertaken because of some evidence that there is immune system disturbance in ALS. Both studies demonstrated no therapeutic benefit.

Cyclosporine and Azathioprine

Two other immune suppressive drugs, cyclosporine (Neoral®) and azathioprine (Imuran®), were also ineffective.

External Irradiation of the Lymph System

More aggressive immunosuppressive therapy was examined utilizing high doses of external irradiation of the lymph system in a controlled trial involving sixty-one patients. This very aggressive trial revealed no therapeutic benefit from radiation therapy.

Interferons

Interferons have been effective in MS, a disease that appears to have a definite immune system component. Interferons have been utilized in several trials in patients with ALS with negative results; however, these trials were quite small (only thirty-seven patients), raising the possibility that further studies might be considered.

Antiviral Agents

Amantadine and Guanidine

A number of studies have raised the possibility that a virus may play a role in developing ALS. Amantadine and guanidine are both drugs that may have a positive effect in combating viruses. These agents were evaluated in

A number of studies have raised the possibility that a virus may play a role in developing ALS.

a controlled trial involving twenty patients in a 6-month trial that showed no benefit.

Isoprinosine

Isoprinosine, another antiviral agent, was examined in two controlled trials involving fifty-eight patients. The results were negative in both studies.

Tilorone

Small trials involving tilorone and α-interferon for an average of only 18 weeks were negative and no beneficial effect was found.

Pleconaril

Pleconaril is a new antiviral agent that appears to be effective against a specific virus (*echo-7*) that seems to have a preferential effect on motor nerves. New evidence suggests that this virus may play a role in the pathogenesis of ALS, although this result is still controversial. Some resolution of this controversy is needed before proceeding to a clinical trial.

Mitochondrial Supporting Agents

Creatine

Recent biochemical and genetic studies suggest that free radical toxicity and impairment of the energy factory of nerve cells, the mitochondria, may be important in ALS. Creatine is a widely available substance that can improve mitochondrial function and has demonstrated neuroprotective capability in an animal model of ALS. Studies of healthy subjects have shown that oral creatine improves maximal exercise performance and the speed of recovery after exercise, as well as increasing the energy available for muscle; however, two large clinical trials in patients with ALS—one in Holland examining survival and one in the United States monitoring strength—were unable to demonstrate a therapeutic benefit of creatine. A third study in the United States is still in progress.

Other Clinical Trials in Progress

Minocycline

A number of clinical trials are in progress at the time of this writing. One of them involves the antibiotic minocycline, which has been used to treat bacterial infections and acne for many years. Very recently, four studies in the ALS mouse model have shown that minocycline can prolong the survival of animals with ALS. The clinical trial in patients with ALS is supported by funds from the NIH and MDA, and involves twenty-four centers across the United States and Canada. The drug has two actions that are relevant to ALS. It can interrupt the final phase of cell death, called *apoptosis* or *preprogrammed cell death*. Proteins that are critical in this pathway are inhibited by minocycline. The drug also blocks the activation of certain cells known as *microglia*, which are important in the immune system activation that occurs in the brain in some patients with ALS. This study was launched in the last quarter of 2003, and it will take 2 to 3 years to get an answer about the effectiveness of minocycline in ALS.

Celecoxib

The nonsteroidal, anti-inflammatory drug celecoxib (Celebrex®) is in a clinical trial in patients with ALS. Celebrex® is approved by the FDA for the treatment of arthritis, but studies suggest that this drug prevents the build-up of glutamate and also the build-up of free radicals in the brain and spinal cord. This drug blocks the action of an enzyme called *cyclo-oxygenase*, which appears to be important in inflammatory processes in the spinal cord and the brain. This enzyme is markedly elevated in patients with ALS, and blocking the enzyme has a beneficial effect on survival in the ALS mouse model. Enrollment in the trial was complete with 300 subjects entered in June 2003. The study was completed in June 2004, with the results expected in the near future.

Tamoxifen

The drug tamoxifen (Nolvadex®), commonly used in the treatment of breast cancer, appeared to slow the rate of decline in a patient with both

ALS and breast cancer. This clinical trial is coordinated at the University of Wisconsin and is currently enrolling a total of 100 subjects. The main measure of effectiveness in the study is the rate of decline of muscular strength.

Indinavir

The drug indinavir (Crixivan®) was recently evaluated in a clinical trial coordinated at Beth Israel Medical Center in New York. This study derived from reports of patients with HIV infection who developed an ALS-like syndrome and responded to high-dose anti-retroviral therapy. This 9-month study was designed to see whether the inhibition of preprogrammed cell death by indinavir can prolong survival for patients with ALS who do *not* have HIV infection. Unfortunately, there was no beneficial effect from indinavir in this trial. The investigators wisely caution patients with ALS not to start treatment with anti-HIV drugs outside of this trial because current studies have only indicated an effect in patients with HIV infection. These patients had unusual features: they were young; they had unusually rapidly progressive weakness; they had a suppressed immune system; and they had evidence of inflammation in the spinal fluid, which is normally absent in patients with ALS without HIV infection.

TCH 346

A new oral compound (TCH 346) developed by Novartis is under study in a clinical trial launched in the third quarter of 2003. This oral agent appears to inhibit preprogrammed cell death and will be studied in four different doses along with placebo. A total of 500 patients were enrolled from 40 centers in North America and Europe. The main measure of effectiveness will be a revised ALS functional rating scale called ALSFRS-R. The medication is administered orally; the study is 13 months in duration.

A 70-year-old man had arm, speech, and swallowing difficulty from ALS. He has been taking riluzole for 6 months and has an opportunity to participate in a placebo-controlled clinical trial of a promising new agent. He wants to know the pros and cons of participating in this kind of clinical research.

Comment: *On the positive side, he has a chance to be on the cutting edge of research for effective treatments for ALS. He might receive an agent that could possibly help him. He has a chance to make a contribution and become partners with a dedicated team that is trying to find effective treatments for ALS. Although there is a risk of side effects from the medication being tested in such trials, there is otherwise relatively little downside from participating in a clinical trial. He will have frequent contact with a research team that is highly knowledgeable about the disease, which should also raise the standard of his care.*

On the downside, he might receive a placebo. If so, there is usually the promise of a period at the end of the study (called an *open-label extension*) wherein it would be guaranteed that he would receive the real thing as a way of saying "thank you" for his participation. This trial would require a fair expenditure of time, and he would have to live with the uncertainty of not knowing whether he was taking placebo or active drug.

Many patients find increased hope through participation in clinical trials, but some are reluctant to take the risk of receiving placebo or experiencing side effects.

Resources

The following resources may be used to obtain information about new and ongoing ALS clinical trials:

- The World Federation of Neurology Web site contains links to other ALS Web sites concerned with ALS Clinical Trials: www.wfn.com
- The ALSA Web site contains information about current clinical trials in ALS: www.alsa.org
- The MDA Web site has current research information about ALS and also listings of current clinical trials: www.als.mdausa.org

- The American Academy of Neurology Web site lists practice guidelines for optimal, evidence-based care of patients with ALS: www.aan.com
- The Cochrane Collaboration Web site is a reliable source of up-to-date information on healthcare and contains evidence-based reviews on ALS: www.cochrane.org/index0.hum

Managing the Symptoms of ALS

CHAPTER 4

A Multidisciplinary Approach to Care

Your choice of a health care provider is a critically important decision. The relationship with your ALS specialist physician will be ongoing

> Your choice of a health care provider is a critically important decision.

and must have a foundation of mutual trust. As you make this decision, you will need to know that your physician will:

- Tell the truth.
- Educate you and your family about the disease.
- Make ongoing assessments.
- Inform you of what to expect in the near and distant future.
- Teach you the skills necessary to alleviate/minimize symptoms.
- Refer you to community support sources.
- Be available for continuing care and support throughout the disease process.
- Inform you of the current treatments available.
- Empower you to make decisions about treatments and interventions that you may or may not accept.
- Intervene in a crisis.

Choosing an ALS Specialist

You need to feel that you can trust your physician to guide you through a myriad of decisions and that you can work effectively with him. The physician who manages the symptoms and course of your disease will function in many ways as the "captain" of a team of professionals. Your ALS specialist physician will interact with your primary care physician, other specialty physicians who may already be involved in your care and those who will be used in the future, a variety of therapists, and a home care team. This specialist will help you to determine when it is the right time to call in other professionals, attempt new directions, recommend standard and experimental treatments, and support your family throughout your disease process. You need to feel that you can have frank and honest discussions with him and that your concerns and priorities are listened and responded to.

Developing the Team

As a result, people with ALS typically need the expertise of doctors who are experienced with the many problems that the disease can produce. You will likely need the services of a neurologist, nurse, physical therapist,

> The needs of a person with ALS are multifaceted and constantly changing.

occupational therapist, speech pathologist, dietitian, respiratory therapist, and social worker. At times, you may also need to be evaluated by a pulmonologist, gastroenterologist, orthotist, and rehabilitation specialist.

The Multidisciplinary Team Approach

The ideal setting for ALS care is a multidisciplinary clinic that specializes in treating patients with ALS and brings all of these specialists together in one place to evaluate your changing and current status. The major advantage of an ALS clinic is that everyone involved has a great deal of experience working with the problems you are likely to encounter and can offer solutions that have worked for others. By offering these services in one location, a clinic can offer a coordinated and well informed plan of care.

Most patients attend ALS clinic every 3 months. You will receive recommendations from the team about the problems you are experiencing at the moment as well as about issues that may be coming up over the next 3 months. This will allow you and your family to make decisions and plan for the changes that you may need to start thinking about.

It can be overwhelming to deal with the technical language that medical professionals use and understand what roles the different team members actually perform. There is a lot of overlap between functions and often there will be two or more therapists working with you on the very same issues. Although clinics are very busy places, you need to become comfortable with asking questions and understanding your treatment plan.

The first few clinic visits can be anxiety-provoking. You may feel that you need to learn a lot but do not even know what questions you want to ask. One way to prepare for your clinic visit is to sit down with family members and list the things in your day-to-day life that cause you problems. It is helpful to organize them by category: walking, dressing, eating, communicating, breathing, and sleeping. Write down your concerns with treatment, your finances, insurance, future planning, and how you and your family are coping. Let your doctor and team members know at the beginning of the visit that you have questions so your concerns will be addressed. Sometimes, there will be more issues than can be addressed in one visit and a follow-up visit can be planned. The team can help you determine what should be your immediate priorities and sort out your concerns.

The Team Players

A description of the roles that team members perform may help you with your question list and in determining who can be the most helpful in solving each problem. You should leave the doctor's office feeling secure that you know how to manage your medication and general care and—if questions remain or arise later—that you know who to contact for follow-up.

Save the list to help you plan for the next visit and to have any unanswered questions addressed.

In some areas, the closest multidisciplinary clinic may be a great distance from where you live. Many patients find it helpful to make the trip less frequently than every 3 months and will follow-up on the recommendations given in their home community. They use the staff at their ALS clinic as a resource to therapists in their local area. If a multidisciplinary clinic is not available, you may want to discuss with your physician how you can obtain assistance from other therapists.

Joe was recently diagnosed with ALS, and he and his wife, Mary, prepared for their first ALS multidisciplinary clinic visit. The following is the problem list they created. The couple shared their list with their ALS specialist doctor.

Walking—Joe finds that he tires more easily and that his toe seems to be catching on the carpet frequently. (Physical Therapist)

Dressing—Joe is capable of dressing without assistance but finds that buttons and shoelaces are becoming more difficult. (Occupational Therapist)

Eating—Eating is no problem, but Joe finds that he sometimes coughs after drinking a glass of water. He has lost 3 pounds in the last 3 months. (Speech Language Pathologist and Nutritionist)

Communication—Early in the day, Joe has no problems, but his speech becomes slurred at about 4:00 in the afternoon. (Speech Language Pathologist)

Breathing—He has no problems breathing, but he is anxious to do everything possible to preserve his breathing muscle strength. (Respiratory Therapist)

Sleeping—Joe finds it difficult to fall asleep because he is worried about work and how to talk with his 8- and 15-year-old children about his diagnosis. (Doctor and Social Worker)

Treatment—*Joe and Mary want to know if they are doing everything possible to help to slow the progress of his disease. (Doctor and Research Coordinator)*

Finances—*Mary and Joe are concerned that Joe's work might be too much for him and that the stress of his job may be speeding up the course of disease. Joe is worried about what will happen to his family financially if he needs to stop working. (Doctor and Social Worker)*

Insurance—*Joe has insurance through his job that covers him and his family, but he worries about what will happen if he cannot continue to work. How will he pay for his upcoming expenses and keep the family covered by insurance? (Social Worker and Nurse)*

Future Planning—*Joe and Mary live in a ranch-style house that has six steps at the entrance. Mary cannot imagine how Joe will manage the stairs if he gets any weaker or needs a wheelchair. (Physical Therapist and Occupational Therapist)*

Coping—*Joe feels like he has his emotions under control, but Mary keeps giving him articles about the disease that make him nervous. Mary feels that Joe is trying to ignore the changes he is experiencing and refuses to plan for the future. They are both worried about how their children will deal with the news. (Doctor and Social Worker)*

Comment: *ALS is a disease that affects the entire family, and there are usually many concerns, both immediate and in the future. Different team members will be of assistance at different times. By presenting all of your current concerns to the doctor and nurse coordinator, they can make certain that your concerns are addressed by the appropriate staff (indicated in parentheses).*

The ALS Specialist Team

The following description of the staff at the ALS clinic will help you understand how each professional can help you.

1. Physician (MD, DO)

The physician's main role is the diagnosis and treatment of ALS and any other underlying disease. You should expect the doctor to explain the diag-

> The physician's main role is the diagnosis and treatment of ALS and any other underlying disease.

nosis and progression of the disease, and to explain the standard and experimental treatments that are available and their potential benefits and side effects.

The physician will help you decide how aggressively you wish to treat symptoms and may refer you to other specialists to help with specific problems that you are experiencing. These specialists may be other physicians or allied professionals, such as nurses and therapists. Your ALS physician will monitor how well you respond to the treatments the specialists recommend.

In addition, your physician will be available to discuss the impact of ALS on your life in general and to help you develop ways to lessen the effect of the disease on your everyday life. Sometimes this can be accomplished with medications or with behavioral or lifestyle changes.

2. Nurse, Nurse Coordinator, Case Manager

The nurse is the coordinator of the multidisciplinary team in most ALS clinics. She will assist you with getting information about your specific problems and coordinate consultations with the therapists and specialists who will treat you both at the clinic and in your home. She will provide information about the management of the disease and explain the terminology, techniques, and procedures. The nurse acts as a resource to other professionals who may be less familiar with the specific problems that people have as a result of their ALS.

In most clinics, the nurse will be available by telephone if you need advice between appointments. She will help you identify and limit the development of complications and will advocate on your behalf to help resolve problems. The nurse can also be a valuable resource in helping you to determine whether the recommended treatments are covered by your insurance.

3. Occupational Therapist (OT)

The occupational therapist is mostly concerned with arm and hand function, and the performance of the *activities of daily living*. She will assess fine motor functional abilities (i.e., hand use) and recommend devices to assist you in performing hygiene, dressing, and eating; managing tasks at home and work; and recreational activities. The OT works closely with the physical therapist to choose equipment for mobility and, if certain equipment (i.e., a wheelchair) is appropriate, the OT will assist you with positioning and seating requirements.

Occupational therapists are concerned with making tasks easier to perform and ways to conserve energy and decrease fatigue. They will recommend splints and exercises to increase hand function and minimize any possible hand and wrist deformity resulting from weakness or stiffness. They will focus on positioning both in bed and while sitting.

The OT works with the speech pathologist to choose the proper device when verbal communication becomes more difficult. He is invaluable in helping families plan for home modifications that will allow for equipment and energy conservation, and can offer resources in the community to assist with modifications.

4. Physical Therapist (PT)

The main focus of the physical therapist is the large muscle groups that coordinate body movements: walking, throwing, balance, and posture.

The PT will analyze and devise ways to optimize walking. He will recommend equipment such as canes, walkers, and wheelchairs, and may advise a brace called an AFO (ankle foot orthosis) to support the foot and make walking easier and safer. The PT can also advise you on equipment for neck and back weakness, and for a droopy head.

The PT will be your main contact for advice on exercise. He will teach you and your family an exercise and stretching program that will maximize your strength and comfort. The PT is also concerned with pain and fatigue. He may recommend other physical treatments (massage, application of heat or cold) that will contribute to comfort and easier movement. The PT also teaches both patients and family members the proper way to move, lift, and transfer without injury. The PT may participate in a home assessment.

5. Respiratory Therapist (RT), Pulmonologist (MD)

The respiratory therapist or pulmonologist focuses on optimizing respiratory muscle function and reducing breathing discomfort. She will evaluate lung function, provide suggestions for maximizing lung function, and may recommend breathing exercises to maintain strength or medications to clear the airways. She will also evaluate the strength of your cough and teach you methods to enhance or compensate for a weakened cough. Suction devices or other equipment may be recommended to loosen secretions and promote airway clearance if secretions are a problem.

She will work with the speech pathologist to provide compensatory techniques for breathing support of nutrition and speech and, when appropriate, will facilitate a home ventilation program.

6. Social Worker, Masters of Social Work (MSW), Licensed Clinical Social Worker (LCSW)

The issues of emotional, social, and environmental problems associated with illness and disability are the main concerns of the social worker. He works to promote an understanding of ALS and assists in adjustment to the disease process. The social worker provides emotional support and helps patients and their families explore coping strategies to enhance communication and understanding within families and their communities. People with ALS often struggle with how to tell children, parents, employers, and friends about their disease; the social worker can be of great assistance in ways to facilitate these discussions.

The social worker will share community resources that can help families contend with problems. He will provide information on legal matters (i.e. advanced directives and living wills) and entitlement programs (i.e., Medicare, Medicaid, and Social Security). The social worker can assist in assigning priorities and making long range plans, such as hiring help in the home.

7. Speech Therapist, Speech-Language Pathologist (SLP)

The speech-language pathologist's concerns are centered around communication and swallowing. She will evaluate speech and swallowing, and evaluate the potential for the person with ALS to learn new techniques of communicating and eating.

One of the primary goals is to offer compensatory techniques and augmentative communication strategies that allow a person to communicate. The speech pathologist will help to determine the most efficient communication techniques at various stages of the disease and train patients and family members in how to use those techniques.

The speech pathologist also evaluates swallowing ability and works closely with the dietitian to recommend the types and consistencies of food that can be safely swallowed.

8. Dietician (RD), Nutritionist, Gastroenterologist (MD)

The dietitian's main concerns are to maintain safe, adequate nutrition and hydration to meet a person's energy requirement. He will make recommendations that will insure balanced nutrition (fluid, calories, and protein), because texture and consistency needs change with increasing difficulty in swallowing. The dietitian works in coordination with a speech pathologist in this regard. The dietitian suggests substitutions for hard-to-manage foods that can boost calories, protein, and fiber; he will also provide information on oral supplements that are commercially available or that can be prepared at home.

A gastroenterologist is a physician who specializes in the treatment of disorders of the gastrointestinal tract. You may be referred to the gastroenterologist if you might benefit from a feeding tube. She will recommend the types of gastrostomy (feeding) tubes that meet your anatomic and lifestyle needs. The nutritionist works in coordination with a gastroenterologist to determine the appropriate amounts and types of nutritional supplementation.

9. Research Coordinator (R.N. Licensed Research Nurse Coordinator)

The research coordinator works closely with the physician who conducts the clinical trials of new experimental therapies, who is also called the *principal investigator*. The research coordinator is generally a nurse but may be any of the professionals listed above. The coordinator will explain available clinical trials to you and then determine if you meet the criteria to participate in these studies. The coordinator is responsible for making sure that all documentation and data collection are performed according to a predetermined protocol. He is responsible for maintaining confidentiality and overseeing the safety of all of the participants in the trial.

10. Additional Members of the Team

Some clinics may have other types of team members or will refer people with ALS to professionals outside their clinic for a variety of needs.

A psychologist or psychiatrist can offer assistance in coping to the person with ALS and family members. She can help sort out and decrease the degree of emotional upheaval that an individual or family is experiencing.

At times, the physical or occupational therapist may refer you to an *orthotist* (bracing specialist), who will design an *orthotic* (brace) to support and align a weak joint. Your therapist might also consult with a rehabilitation specialist who designs and supplies equipment, such as wheelchairs, that will help you in your home.

Advantages and Disadvantages of a Multidisciplinary Clinic

The multidisciplinary clinic offers many advantages, but it also has some drawbacks. Clinic appointments are long, often lasting over 3 hours; this can be tiring, especially if you must travel long distances to get there. A lot of information is given in a short period of time, and some of it may come before you are emotionally prepared to deal with it. There may be so much information that it is difficult to process. The visit can be expensive because of the breadth of service and the number of professionals involved, although generally costs are covered by insurance or other third-party payors, including the Muscular Dystrophy Association.

Evidence-Based Medicine in Managing ALS

One of the major new guiding principles for managing ALS has come from the emergence of *evidence-based guidelines* in the arena of health care. The goal of evidence-based practice guidelines is to raise the standard of care for all patients and to standardize the way in which different practitioners administer care. Before the advent of evidence-based medicine, many treatment strategies were based on lessons learned in training of the physician,

> The goal of evidence-based practice guidelines is to raise the standard of care for all patients.

personal opinion, recent articles, or discussions with experts. As a result, there has been a substantial variation in treatment practices between different physicians and also between specialized care centers. This is true in ALS management as well as in general medical treatment. One example of this high degree of variance is the pattern of utilization of noninvasive positive pressure mechanical ventilation (NPPV) for patients with breathing difficulties. In one large North American study, utilization of NPPV ranged from 0 to 50 percent of patients in different clinics.

Evidence-based medicine offers a new way to make decisions about medical treatment and provides a solid basis for decision-making in managing ALS. In the evidence-based medicine process, all pertinent studies are analyzed, the evidence is examined, and recommendations are formulated to guide clinical decision-making. The resultant analysis of all available studies provides an evidence-based guideline for managing a disease like ALS.

Recently, the American Academy of Neurology (AAN) sponsored an evidence-based review of management strategies for patients with ALS. The purpose of this review was to improve standards of medical care and quality of life.

A multidisciplinary task force identified 750 relevant articles that met predetermined criteria. The details of the literature search, a more complete description of the process, and a more detailed summary of the evidence are described in the medical literature.

The following principles of managing patients with ALS were agreed upon by the task force:

1. Respect for patient decision-making
2. The importance of informing patients within their cultural and personal context
3. Attention to appropriate timing for decision-making, which may change over time
4. The importance of providing the full spectrum of care from diagnosis through palliative care in the terminal phase

Evidence gleaned from the world's literature pertinent to ALS management was classified, and recommendations for management were developed based on the existing evidence. The guidelines for ALS management were focused on five areas:

1. Informing patients about the diagnosis and future course of the disease
2. Symptomatic treatment

3. Nutrition and feeding tubes
4. Managing breathing issues
5. *Palliative care*, aimed at improving comfort and preserving quality of life

The issues that were developed about sharing the news of a diagnosis of ALS were discussed in the first two chapters. The focus here is how to give the news in a candid and clear fashion, but in a way that preserves some hope. Information about symptomatic treatment is discussed in Chapter 6; issues about swallowing and nutrition are developed in Chapter 7; guidelines for managing breathing issues are listed in Chapter 8; and the recommendations for palliative care, which are designed to enhance comfort and dignity as well as quality of life, are discussed in Chapter 12.

The Good and Bad News about Evidence-Based ALS Management Guidelines

The good news is that the analysis of all of the available evidence from the world's literature about ALS has yielded clear-cut guidelines that can raise the standard of care and improve the treatment of persons with ALS. The

> A steadily increasing number of patients are receiving care that is consistent with the evidence-based practice guidelines.

bad news is that the utilization of these evidence-based guidelines is still not universal. Barriers to implementation of the guidelines include a number of factors: some physicians are not aware of the guidelines; others may not agree with some of them; third-party payer policies and limited financial resources may limit implementation; and not all patients willingly accept the evidence-based recommendations.

A steadily increasing number of patients are receiving care that is consistent with the evidence-based practice guidelines. Nonetheless, a significant percentage of patients still do not receive ideal nutritional, breathing, and palliative care.

One of the major goals of this book is to familiarize you and your family with the evidence-based ALS management guidelines. The guidelines that are pertinent to each of the sections mentioned above will be outlined in detail in the appropriate chapters. We urge you to become a knowledgeable health care consumer, and to advocate with your health care providers to ensure that you receive the high standard of care described in the ALS practice guidelines. The guidelines concerning nutrition and breathing issues are particularly important because they not only *prolong* life but they also raise the *quality* of life. Each of these interventions is at least as powerful as the one available drug, riluzole, which does prolong life but does not enhance its quality. Similarly, the practice guidelines regarding palliative care are critically important for preserving comfort, dignity, and quality of life in the advanced stages of the disease. We urge you to ensure that you understand these issues and that you receive care from experts who provide full access to the high standards of care recommended in the practice guidelines.

Supporting You through the Process

A new diagnosis of ALS can be overwhelming, but many individuals will support you and your family through the process. An ongoing partnership with caregivers can provide families with the tools to maintain a good quality of life. You should expect to learn how to manage symptoms and receive straightforward information about the disease. Your health care team should provide you with ongoing counseling about adapting to changes over time and empower you to make the decisions that are right for you and your family.

CHAPTER 5

Quality of Life and Psychosocial Issues

This chapter deals with the wide variety of factors—both positive and negative—that contribute to quality of life. Much has been written and published about the factors that contribute to maintaining a good quality of life. Some aspects of quality of life that contribute to well-being and a

> Some aspects of quality of life are still largely a mystery.

sense of having a good life worth living are still largely a mystery, such as sexuality and spirituality. Some of the aspects of living with a chronic disease have not been adequately addressed in the ALS literature, although it is increasingly apparent that this is extremely important to people with the disease and their families. This chapter will review what we know as well as those areas that, to date, have been little studied.

Health is defined by the World Health Organization as "a state of complete physical, mental, and social well-being and not merely the absence of disease or infirmity." As health is described in these *holistic* terms, so too must illness be described. There is increasing consensus that the personal burden of ALS cannot be described fully by measures of disease severity, such as muscle strength testing, functional rating scales, breathing capacity, or length of survival. Psychosocial factors, including dependency on others, financial burdens, and the inability to fulfill personal and professional roles, must also be included by any meaningful disease measurement to better understand the various effects that ALS and the treatment of ALS have on daily life and personal satisfaction. Age and family status can also profoundly affect the impact of the disease on a person's life.

For example, the same severity of paralysis in ALS may be expected to have widely varying impacts on a 35-year-old man with a young family and financial responsibilities versus a 65-year-old retired widower in an assisted living facility.

People diagnosed with ALS know that they have a progressive disease with no known cure. Some are able to live the remainder of their lives fully and productively; others are not. Quality of life is not determined solely by disease severity, but rather it seems to be more closely related to other variables, such as optimism and spirituality, which are only poorly understood. Many studies have evaluated quality of life in ALS, but there is no agreement as to what constitutes quality of life and no good way to measure it. Also, because quality of life itself is so individual, it is difficult if not impossible to compare quality of life from one person to another.

The Importance of Measuring Quality of Life

In recent years, there has been an increasing interest in understanding the effects of ALS, and its potential treatments, not only on *quantity* of life (survival), but also *quality* of life. In part, this interest is driven by increasing patient education, the rising cost of health care, the costs of nontraditional and alternative treatments, and the impact of these interventions on outcomes that are valued by the patient. However, the more important reason for understanding the effects of ALS on quality of life is the positive effect that a good quality of life has on survival in this still incurable disease.

The need for quality as well as quantity of life information about treatments in ALS is very evident in the dilemma that many patients face as to whether to take riluzole (Rilutek®), the only disease-specific treatment for ALS. Riluzole modestly extends survival in ALS; however, at a cost of approximately $800 U.S. dollars a month, the difficult question is whether riluzole is of sufficient value to the patient to justify the expense, especially if that expense is to be paid out-of-pocket. There are no data to answer this question because no quality of life measures were incorporated into the original riluzole research trials. One study suggests that patients taking riluzole stay in a milder disease state for a longer period of time. (These issues regarding riluzole were discussed in more detail in Chapter 3.) Ideally, quality of life measures should be incorporated into all ALS treatment trials. However, no ALS-specific measurement tool presently exists and, thus, there is no "gold standard." Some specific recommendations of the World Federation of Neurology with regard to measurement of quality of life in research trials are:

1. Quality of life cannot be used as the only outcome measure at this time, because it is such an individual measure and good quality to one patient may not be good quality to another.
2. More ALS-specific and quality of life scales are needed that are sensitive to the changes caused by the disease.
3. The quality of life of caregivers should also be measured during research trials.
4. Factors that affect quality of life, such as depression, should also be measured because they may be treatable and can influence patient survival.

Physicians would be better able to compare severity of disease states and influence public policy and health care dollars in ways that matter most to patients if good quality of life data were incorporated into research trials.

Assessing Quality of Life

The difficulty in measuring the effects of ALS on the psychosocial aspects of a patient's life is that quality of life tends to be defined in terms of physical function; it focuses on what people can or cannot do. Yet, for most of us, good health is not the end to which we aspire as human beings; it is a means of achieving that end. To assign a value to quality of life, we must first identify what it is that makes life worth living. Quality of life in ALS, as in any disease, is subjective and can only be determined by asking the patient. Outside observers cannot judge a patient's quality of life, and they consistently underestimate the quality of life of patients with disabilities. Quality of life can only be described in individual terms; it is dependent on past experiences, present lifestyle, and future hopes. It also changes with time and circumstances. A good quality of life is said to be present when the hopes of a person are matched and fulfilled by experience. In order to improve quality of life, the gap between one's hopes and what actually occurs must narrow.

> *After 2 years of ALS, a 50-year-old woman has accepted the limitations imposed by her disease. She no longer judges her life in terms of her professional productivity, her tennis game, or her figure. She now enjoys her morning routine with caregivers and daily visits with friends. She is especially looking forward to her oldest daughter's upcoming wedding. Although initially very upset and depressed after receiving the diagnosis of ALS, 2 years later she has adjusted and—as a result of lowering her expectations—again derives a great deal of satisfaction from her life.*

This concept helps explain many apparent paradoxes in life, such as why a beautiful, young movie star like Marilyn Monroe could seemingly "have it all" and yet internally not achieve the measure of success that she sought and decide that life was not worth living, while a young girl paralyzed after surviving a near fatal car accident could feel very grateful for a second chance at life. Quality of life may be improved either by improving present reality or by decreasing expectations (i.e., making the goals more realistic). This helps explain how some patients with ALS are able to have a good quality of life despite severe physical disability. The ability of some people to sustain quality of life despite severe disease has been repeatedly described in the medical literature. One study that evaluated seven ventilator-dependent patients with ALS who were totally bedridden and had no ability to speak or to eat by mouth, and who seldom left their beds, found that none of those patients regretted the decision to go on a ventilator and that most felt contented and satisfied a majority of the time. As changes in health occur, life takes on a new form; it narrows, sometimes to a single room, a single bed. Values change such that what was once important may seem inconsequential, while things once ignored take on new significance. In reality, disease may detract from, enhance, or have no effect upon quality of life.

Quality of life is dynamic and changes over time, yet individuals have personal qualities, such as optimism and coping skills, which help define

> Quality of life is dynamic and changes over time.

their new "set point." These psychological variables determine the way a given individual will perceive himself, his life circumstance, and the correctability of various problems that inhibit personal happiness. Patients who are better able to attach meaning to events such as illness are better able to seek out information and are better able to cope with disease. Ultimately, some individuals are simply more prone to happiness and optimism due to unknown genetic, psychological, and environmental factors.

An 80-year-old married man was recently diagnosed with ALS. His wife of 55 years is alive and well. His adult children live nearby and visit him frequently. Although he can no longer walk, he is taken out daily in his wheelchair and is always accompanied by a loved one. He has no physical pain. His brother died 1 year ago of a painful cancer. He had always suspected that he would die in a similar manner. He is satisfied with what he has accomplished in life, and his reality—a slow painless death from ALS—is better than his expectation of a painful death from cancer. His quality of life is good.

Individuals who have a greater capacity to adapt their expectations to the demands of ALS and set reasonable goals have a greater capacity for life fulfillment and feel less hopeless. Patients may set some expectations that are unrealistically high (a form of denial) or unacceptably low (a form of detachment), yet patients form these expectations by their interpretation of the world around them and are subsequently contented or miserable. The physician who helps the patient accept the disease by setting attainable expectations is as much a healer as the one who can improve reality by improving the patient's physical condition. By understanding the patient's hopes and expectations, the physician and other health care team members may suggest management that will help better achieve patient goals.

A 45-year-old man with a diagnosis of ALS ardently desired to see his son graduate from high school. The patient's breathing capacity was very limited, and he was continually choking on his own saliva due to weakness in his swallowing muscles. Although long-term tracheostomy-ventilatory support imposed great financial hardship on the patient and his new wife, his desire to see his only child graduate was his main goal in life. The decision was therefore made to undergo tracheostomy, and the patient was on full ventilator support as he proudly witnessed his son's commencement ceremony. A local television network interviewed father and son as a human interest story. One month later, the patient requested to be disconnected from the ventilator and this request was respected. He was allowed to die with comfort and dignity.

Emerging evidence suggests that improving quality of life can also prolong life. Although ALS is a relentlessly progressive paralyzing disease with no known cause or cure, and death is inevitable, the course of the disease and length of survival is highly variable. Natural history studies in ALS report that more than 20 percent of patients will survive for 5 years or longer. In a large study of 144 people with ALS, psychological resiliency, spirituality, and psychological well-being were all predictive of long-term survival. In this study, patients with high psychological distress had a seven-fold greater risk of death than patients with enhanced psychological well-being. These data suggest that improvement in psychological well-being extends survival time in ALS.

Hope and the Ability to Cope

Other factors may be involved in quality of life and the ability to cope effectively with ALS. The pace of progression of ALS varies greatly, and in some instances, the spread of weakness seems to occur more rapidly than

> The pace of progression of ALS varies greatly.

the person with ALS can emotionally keep up with. In other people, the spread of weakness is relatively slow and patients appear to be able to adjust their expectations and make appropriate decisions to cope as their disability increases. A theory has been proposed to explain how hope is challenged by the trauma of devastating illness:

1. Initially, at the time of diagnosis, emotions are suspended and all of the person's energy is invested in trying to "hold it all together." All effort is directed at remaining in control. There is no real conscious processing of the meaning of the diagnosis. Emotions are suppressed.

2. In the next stage, the patient is ready to recognize the trauma that has occurred. A goal is identified, which is to get well; however, a means to achieving that goal is not known. This is a time of some uncertainty. People with ALS may seek one medical opinion after another during this period, hoping to find an expert who can provide the missing knowledge of how to return to health. Others may enroll in research trials in the belief that through research, a return to health will eventually be achieved. This stage of sustained hope can be maintained indefinitely, even as people enter the final stages of disease and hospice care.

3. As the weakness of ALS increases and the patient begins to acknowledge the reality of the disease, the period of uncertainty is gone and emotional suffering begins with despair and hopelessness. In this period of blackness, patients seek comfort from others and from their spiritual beliefs; they often become active in ALS support groups. They begin to move away from the past and piece together a new

future based on acceptance of the disease. Thus, suffering can be seen as a way of beginning to heal. At this stage, patients are often able to provide support to those who are newly diagnosed.

4. Finally, the acceptance achieved through suffering transforms into a new hope based in the realistic assessment of the threat that the diagnosis of ALS presents. A path toward a goal is identified, although the outcome is not certain. Emotions are held in check during this stage, as disappointments are anticipated. The person will usually seek supportive relationships at this stage, which are essential for maintaining hope.

Caregivers

The caregiver is an often overlooked but indispensable member of the care team. Four general themes are common among caregivers:

1. Powerlessness over ALS
2. Guilt over not doing enough for their loved one
3. Resentment over unappreciated and unrecognized efforts in caregiving
4. Lack of time to pursue personal interests

Distress in caregivers is associated more with loss of intimacy with the patient than the patient's increased level of disability. Levels of psychic distress (suffering, hopelessness, worry, or depression) in the person with ALS are often very similar to those of the caregiver. Patients worry about the well-being of their caregivers, who are often exhausted, even though caregivers feel fulfilled by the care they minister to patients. They also frequently neglect their own health problems. The well-being of caregivers should be monitored during ALS center visits, in addition to that of the person with ALS, to assure maximal quality of life for the patient.

Sexuality

More than any other topic, the importance of sexuality in ALS remains undiscussed. In a recent U.S. poll of 500 healthy people over age 25, 94 percent felt that a satisfying sex life was an important component of quality of life, although 71 percent said they felt their doctors would dismiss any concerns raised about sexual problems. Sixty-eight percent felt that discussing sexuality would embarrass their physicians, but 85 percent indicated they would discuss sexual problems with their physicians even though they might not receive any help. Patients with ALS—who may be suffering from depression, anxiety, and overwhelming fatigue—may also find that they

> More than any other topic, the importance of sexuality in ALS remains undiscussed.

have a loss of libido. In addition, those with diminished respiratory function would be expected to have less energy available for sexual relations. Your health care team should provide instruction in less strenuous positions such as side-lying, as well as the importance of planning sexual encounters for when you are rested. Many of the drugs used in the treatment of ALS symptoms, in particular those used to treat excess saliva and depression, cause difficulty with sustaining an erection. As with any other medical problem, you should feel free to discuss sexual problems and side effects of medications with your doctor in order to work out a plan of management. Most physicians see sexuality as an important area for medical intervention. An excellent reference is *Sexual Function in People with Disability and Chronic Illness: a Health Professional's Guide* by Sipski M.L. and Alexander C.J. Gaithersburg, Maryland: Aspen Publishers, 1997.

Spirituality

Today, the public understanding of spirituality has evolved and is no longer seen solely in the traditional framework of a relationship with God or a Greater Power, but in the personal and psychological search for meaning in one's life.

Spirituality and the sustaining value of religious conviction benefit the person with ALS by providing a set of core beliefs about life and an ethical foundation for decision-making. In both Oregon and the Netherlands, where assisted suicide is legal, ALS patients with strong religious beliefs are less likely to consider this option. Religious belief provides a constant source of strength that helps buffer the changes of ALS. Most ALS health care providers are willing to engage in a personal dialogue about religion and spirituality. If your health care providers do not initiate the conversation, do not hesitate to start this dialogue yourself if you desire to discuss your search for answers to the ultimate questions of life, death, and suffering.

CHAPTER 6

Treating the Symptoms of ALS

People with ALS frequently complain that, after giving them the diagnosis, their doctors do not want to see them, do not want to talk to them, and do not know how to comfort them. In fact, many physicians may feel powerless in managing a person with ALS. The important point is that, although ALS cannot be cured, it *can* be effectively treated. In this chapter, we will discuss both medications to slow the progression of the disease and also the treatment of specific symptoms. If you receive your care at an ALS clinic, these treatments will be familiar to your physician and he will inform you of ways in which he can help you cope with your disease. If you receive your ALS care from a community physician, this chapter might be useful to share with your treating physician, as it may provide him with ideas as to how better to help you manage your illness. You have the right to expect your doctor to take the time to become informed about your specific problems with ALS. At each appointment, you have the opportunity to teach your physician more about ALS and how it affects you. Your physician has the responsibility to help prepare you for the future so that the impact of the disease on your life will be lessened.

Treatment to Slow the Progression of ALS

People with ALS are primarily interested in pursuing treatment once the diagnosis of ALS has been established. The only specific treatment for ALS that is approved by the U.S. Food and Drug Administration (FDA) at this time is riluzole (Rilutek®). Two large placebo-controlled double-blind trials demonstrated that riluzole modestly extends survival for people with ALS (see Chapter 3). Further analysis of the data suggested that patients treated with riluzole stayed in milder ALS disease states longer than patients who were not treated.

Treating Specific Symptoms

Table 6-1 summarizes the medications commonly used to treat the symptoms of ALS.

Weakness

Although the progressive weakness of ALS cannot be stopped or reversed, there are adaptive strategies. Occupational and physical therapists can provide numerous assistive devices to help with feeding, dressing, walking, and other activities of daily living (see Chapters 4 and 9).

Muscle Aches, Cramps, and Spasms

A muscle cramp is a sudden, unintended muscle contraction that may occur in the arms, legs, chest, back, abdomen, jaw, or throat. Cramps are caused by overstimulation of the nerves of a weakened muscle. These contractions may be extremely painful and prolonged. You may experience knotting in the muscle and abnormal posture until the cramp passes. You can help manage cramps by maintaining a proper diet, drinking plenty of water, and avoiding overexertion of your weaker muscles. Stretching is also a very effective way of stopping a muscle cramp. Medication can be prescribed when cramps are particularly frequent and severe.

Spasticity

Spasticity is a change in the *resting tone* of your muscles that leaves them feeling tight and stiff. The legs become difficult to bend, and walking becomes unbalanced and slow when spasticity is severe. The legs will not relax when sitting and will have a tendency to straighten at the knee. This stiff feeling can make it difficult to fall asleep at night and remain comfortable throughout the night. Many medications are available to relax this

TABLE 6-1

Commonly Used Medications for Symptomatic ALS Treatment

Symptom	Medication
Muscle cramps and spasms	Baclofen, tizanidine (Zanaflex®), quinine sulfate (quinine)
Excessive laughter or crying	Tricyclic antidepressants (Amitriptyline®), selective serotonin reuptake inhibitors (Lexapro®, Celexa®, Zoloft®, Prozac®) valproate (Depakote®), lithium (Lithobid®)
Spasticity (stiffness of limbs)	Baclofen, tizanidine (Zanaflex®), benzodiazepines (Valium®)
Urinary urgency or frequency	Oxybutynin (Ditropan®)
Excessive saliva	Tricyclic antidepressants (Amitriptyline®), glycopyrrolate (Robinul®), scopolamine (TransDerm®), botulinum toxin injection (Botox®)
Thick phlegm/postnasal drip	Guaifenesin (Robitussin®, Humibid®), nebulizer treatments
Laryngospasm (throat-closing spasm)	Benzodiazepines (Valium®, Klonapin®, Ativan®)
Jaw quivering/clenching of the teeth	Benzodiazepines (Valium®, Klonapin®, Ativan®)
Nasal congestion	Steroid nasal spray (Beconase®, Nasonex®)
Acid reflux	Omeprazole (Prilosec®), famotidine (Pepcid®), ranitidine (Zantac®), cimetidine (Tagamet®), metoclopromide (Reglan®)
Insomnia	Tricyclic antidepressants (Trazodone®), zolpidem (Ambien®), temazepam (Restoril®)
Depression/anxiety	Selective serotonin reuptake inhibitors (Prozac®, Paxil®, Zoloft®, Celexa®, Lexapro®), venlafaxine (Effexor®), bupropion (Welbutrin®), mirtazapine (Remeron®)
Shortness of breath	Morphine elixir
Pain	Nonsteroidal anti-inflammatory (Motrin®, Celebrex®, Vioxx®), pain medication (Tylenol®, Darvon®, aspirin), narcotics (Vicodin®, morphine, Oxycontin®)
Nausea	THC (Marinol®), prochlorperazine (Compazine®)
Constipation	Stool softeners (Colace®), laxatives (Senekot®, Ducolax®), fiber (Metamucil®), enemas
Agitation/anxiety	Benzodiazepines (Ativan®, Xanax®, Valium®)
Terminal agitation	Morphine, atypical neuroleptics (Seroquel®, Zyprexa®), thorazine (Thioridazine®) (if sedation desired)

increased muscle tone or stiffness and restore muscles to a more natural state. Care must be taken not to use high doses of these medications, because excessive muscle relaxation or weakness could result.

Fatigue

Generalized fatigue and exhaustion are common features of ALS. As nerve cells die, the remaining ones send signals to activate the otherwise unused muscle and a single surviving nerve cell may be doing a hundred times its normal workload. This may result in temporary exhaustion of overworked nerve cells. Thus, there may be times when you can perform a task, such as climbing stairs, only when you have rested beforehand. You should pace yourself wisely in terms of energy expenditure throughout the day and the week. Various medications have been tried for fatigue with little success and are therefore not recommended. When persistent overwhelming fatigue is a problem, your quality of sleep should be evaluated, because ineffective sleep and also depression are common causes of daytime fatigue.

Sleep Disturbance

Sleep disturbance can erode quality of life and cause other difficulties, such as depression and fatigue. Many factors can contribute to an inability to sleep. Sleep disorders in ALS may result from depression and anxiety, as well as nighttime breathing disturbances due to sleep apnea or weakened breathing muscles (see Chapter 10). If you are not sleeping well, you and your doctor should try to determine why. The cause could vary from simple insomnia to anxiety and depression or breathing problems. The best treatment for problems with sleep will be the one that gets at the specific problem that prevents you from sleeping.

Excessive Laughter or Crying

People with ALS sometimes develop difficulty controlling their emotions and will cry or laugh inappropriately or excessively. This is thought to be caused by the loss of motor control over the brain centers involved in laughing and crying. These symptoms are embarrassing and they are often not recognized as being part of ALS. Antidepressants and the other medications listed in Table 6-1 are effective in treating these unwanted displays of emotion.

Urinary Urgency or Frequency

Although ALS usually does not involve the bladder muscles in the early phases, people with ALS frequently develop an irritable bladder with urinary urgency and frequency. This may be due to the loss of motor control over the brain centers for urination. In addition, urinary tract infections will also increase bladder spasms and frequency of urination. Therefore, when there is a marked increase in urinary frequency, an analysis of a urine sample should be performed, and any infection should be treated with antibiotics. In men, the prostate gland may be enlarged, resulting in the need to urinate frequently. Medication may be helpful to relax the bladder and lessen urinary symptoms if no infection is present.

Swelling of Hands and Feet

Swelling frequently occurs in a very weak limb due to failure of the muscle pumping action that increases blood return to the heart. Passive range of motion, elevation of paralyzed limbs, and compression hose are helpful. When swelling in one leg is painful or fails to decrease after overnight elevation, a blood clot or deep vein thrombosis (DVT) should be suspected and evaluated immediately because of the risk of the clot traveling to the lungs (pulmonary embolism). You should discuss blood clot prevention with your physician prior to prolonged periods of inactivity, such as airplane travel.

Excessive Salivation

Excessive saliva, a common feature of ALS, results in increased drooling, choking, or coughing. The problem is not due to overproduction of saliva, but to decreased swallowing. Saliva is not swallowed automatically by those with ALS, and you must consciously swallow saliva to compensate for this. Excess saliva may be further increased by anxiety, hunger, and acid reflux. There are many medications to decrease saliva (see Table 6-1, page 93), and you can request them from your physician. Surgery and radiotherapy have both been tried for excess secretions but often result in excessively thickened secretions. Botulinum toxin (Botox®) injections into the salivary glands have very effectively reduced excess saliva in many people with ALS when medications are no longer effective. This treatment lasts for approximately 3 months and may be repeated when needed.

Thick Phlegm/Postnasal Drip

People with ALS may develop the habit of breathing through the mouth because of fatigue of the jaw muscles or nasal congestion. Breathing through the mouth causes the saliva to dry out and thicken. Furthermore, medications taken to reduce drooling can cause excessive dryness and thick secretions, which can result in postnasal drip, chronic cough, or a need to clear the throat. Certain medications have been reported to thin secretions when added to antisaliva regimens. Nonprescription cough syrups may be helpful in thinning saliva. Chicken broth and hot tea, as well as the use of room humidifiers, oral suction machines, and aerosolized breathing treatments can also help. When allergies contribute to postnasal drip, antihistamines and steroid nasal inhalers may also be useful.

Jaw Quivering and Clenching of the Teeth

Some people with ALS may experience an uncomfortable tightening or chattering of the jaw due to cold, anxiety, or pain. Medications may be helpful in relieving these symptoms as well.

Laryngospasm (Tightening of the Throat)

Laryngospasm is an abrupt and prolonged closure of the vocal cords resulting in sudden gasping for breath and wheezing. This can cause panic because of the fear of suffocation. Laryngospasm may also occur with increased emotion or with exposure to smoke, strong smells, alcohol, cold or rapid bursts of air, and even spicy foods. It can also occur with sinus or postnasal drip, as well as acid reflux. Laryngospasm normally clears spontaneously in a few seconds, but can be more immediately relieved by breathing through the nose and repetitively swallowing. Possible triggers of laryngospasm should be eliminated and a trial of antacids instituted. Understanding the nature of this process can usually help to calm the panic that aggravates laryngospasm.

Acid Reflux

Acid reflux, also known as gastroesophageal reflux disease (GERD), is a common condition in people with ALS. It is due to weakness of the diaphragm muscles involved in breathing, which normally form a tight band around the opening to the stomach to keep the acids down. The signs and symptoms may include heartburn, acid taste, throat irritation, chest pain, hoarseness, shortness of breath, nausea, insomnia, and even spasms of the larynx. These symptoms are thought to be caused by the reflux of stomach acid into the lower esophagus. Caffeine, spicy foods, overeating, and diaphragm weakness all increase acid reflux into the esophagus. Particular care in managing this problem is necessary if a feeding tube is used because the stomach may be easily overfilled. Medications to increase clearance of foods from the stomach (metoclopramide) as well as antacids (ranitidine hydrochloride, cimetidine, famotidine, and omeprazole) are quite effective.

Nasal Congestion

The muscles in the nose and mouth may be weakened, resulting in a failure to elevate and open the nostrils, the upper airways, and the Eustacian tubes, which connect to the ears. The nasal airways can be opened effectively by applying nasal tape across the bridge of the nose to open nasal passages, as used by athletes. Steroid nasal sprays take several days to take effect but can be very helpful in relieving congestion.

Constipation

Constipation is common in ALS and, if untreated, can result in hours spent on the toilet with abdominal pain and bloating. Constipation in ALS is caused by decreased fluid, inadequate diet, lack of exercise, and a reduced ability to bear down with the abdominal muscles. Proper management is essential because hospitalization for bowel obstruction may be necessary if this condition persists. Medications taken to control excessive saliva and pain can contribute to constipation and should be decreased if possible or discontinued when not necessary. An excellent dietary recipe to normalize bowel movement is "power pudding," which consists of equal parts of prunes, prune juice, applesauce, and bran. Two tablespoons with each meal and at bedtime, along with adequate fluid intake and fruits and vegetables in the diet, helps in maintaining normal bowel movements. Stool softeners, laxatives, and periodic enemas should be used liberally, when necessary.

Depression and Anxiety

Depression is common in anyone with increasing physical disability and should be aggressively treated. Depression is underdiagnosed and undertreated in ALS, and it has a negative effect on the quality of life of both patients and their families. Newer antidepressants (the selective serotonin reuptake inhibitors) are preferable to the older types of antidepressants (such as amitriptyline) because of their greater efficacy and lesser side effects. When effective, antidepressants should be continued for at least 6 months to one year and then slowly tapered as indicated. Buspirone and benzodiazepines can be used on an as-needed basis when anxiety and agitation are the main problems. Buspirone is preferable because it does not suppress the muscles involved in breathing.

Difficulty in Swallowing

Weakness and incoordination of the mouth and throat muscles can result in swallowing problems. A swallowing evaluation by a speech therapist can be helpful in determining which foods cause the greatest difficulty (see

Chapter 7). For mild swallowing problems, you should tuck your chin down, swallow two to three times per mouthful of food, avoid foods that cause the greatest difficulty, and perform a clearing cough after each swallow. When swallowing difficulty results in weight loss or when a patient becomes fatigued in attempts to consume a meal, a percutaneous gastrostomy (PEG) should be considered. The procedure should be carried out before excess weight loss occurs and while the patient has good breathing function, because the risk of complications increases in weaker patients. They should be fed only in an upright position and should avoid bending or lying flat for at least 1 hour after eating, to prevent food from entering the lungs. In many instances, medicines such as metoclopramide may be added to aid emptying of the stomach. Most people with a PEG prefer feedings at regular mealtimes to leave time available for other activities. A variety of feeding formulas are available. In general, concentrated formulas with high fat and sugar content are harder to digest and may result in cramping and diarrhea. Less concentrated solutions are preferable and may be specifically selected to meet individual needs (i.e., high-fiber formulas for constipation; high protein, high lipid, low carbohydrate formulas for patients with shortness of breath) (see Chapter 7).

Slurred Speech

Slurred, slow, or strangulated speech is caused by incoordination and weakness of the lips, tongue, and throat muscles. People with speech problems should be evaluated by a speech therapist and alternative communication methods explored (see Chapter 8). Some form of communication can usually be established and must be sought. It is essential that the family members recognize and respect the patient's need to communicate, even when it is time-consuming and frustrating.

Shortness of Breath

Breathing problems may arise from many different causes in ALS. For this reason, breathing difficulties should be evaluated by a physician familiar with both breathing problems and ALS (see Chapter 10).

Pain and Pressure Sores

Although pain is not generally thought to be a feature of ALS, it is extremely common late in the course of disease. Pain may be due to muscle cramping or joint changes such as hip dislocation. Pain can also occur when there is prolonged immobility of paralyzed limbs, such as when a caregiver is not available to reposition the person frequently. A pressure sore may develop if the body has been in the same position for many hours. Pressure sores are particularly apt to develop over bony areas, such as the tip of the spine. Alternating airflow mattresses and air and gel cushions can reduce pressure over these tender spots. Mild pain associated with pressure sores may be relieved by ibuprofen or acetaminophen, but narcotic medications may be needed for more severe pain.

Alternative Treatment

People with ALS are often dissatisfied (as are their physicians) with the specific treatment offered by conventional medicine to slow the disease process and many patients seek alternative solutions to their disease. These holistic approaches may benefit the patient greatly in affording a sense of mastery over the disease. Nutritional regimens that stress the role of antioxidant vitamins in postponing symptom manifestation have some basis in research. Vitamin E treatment has been shown to delay the onset of symptoms in a mouse model of ALS, although it did not have an impact on survival. It has now become common to recommend 2,000 I.U. of vitamin E per day in combination with riluzole as a treatment for ALS. Milk or some other form of fat in the stomach greatly enhances the absorption of vitamin E.

Other holistic remedies have not been proven valuable; however, other approaches, such as therapeutic massage and visual imagery, may offer support, encouragement, and hope. None of us can live without hope, and people with ALS should be encouraged to share their exploration into alternative treatments with their physicians. The physician should serve as an advisor, steering patients away from harmful therapies and towards those that may help. For those who desire a holistic approach, it is important to find an ALS physician who is willing to communicate with alternative medicine providers so that your overall ALS treatment can be coordinated and beneficial. In this way, you will feel free to ask for more conventional therapies when the need arises. Ultimately, it is your decision as to how your disease will be treated.

Terminal Management

At some point in the progression of ALS, you may become tired of the struggle to continue living. Many people with ALS ultimately reach a level where they feel they can no longer maintain a satisfactory quality of life. At this point, the emphasis shifts from extending life to making the remaining days more comfortable (see Chapter 12). Nursing agencies can arrange home visits when you find it too difficult to go to the clinic for periodic evaluation. Most people desire to be pain-free at this point in the disease; they want to be as alert as possible during the day and have a comfortable, uninterrupted night's sleep. They should be given whatever treatment is necessary to relieve suffering, even if it does shorten life. Antianxiety medications (lorazepam), sleeping pills (temazepam), and pain relievers (including morphine) should be available as needed. People with ALS sometimes may require antinausea medications (prochlorperazene), because both shortness of breath and the medications to relieve it may cause stomach upset. Most people are reassured by the knowledge that their death will be peaceful and without struggle, lack of air, or pain.

Quality of Life

Although no one would ever choose to have ALS, many people with the disease affirm that ALS has brought blessings as well as suffering. They report new appreciation of family, friends, the beauty of nature, and life itself. Many people find the capacity to enjoy life each and every day. Morrie Schwartz, who had ALS, wrote, "After you have wept and grieved for your physical losses, cherish the functions and life that you have left." As health care providers, we consider it a privilege to be included in this intimate celebration of living and witness how ordinary people summon extraordinary faith and courage to overcome the hardships imposed by ALS and continue to live full lives.

CHAPTER 7

Nutrition and Swallowing

Alycia Chu, MS, RD

Maintaining good nutrition is one of the greatest challenges of living with ALS. It may become increasingly difficult for you to take in adequate calories and protein. This is often seen when there is difficulty chewing and swallowing, becoming full quickly and easily fatigued, taste

> Maintaining good nutrition is one of the greatest challenges of living with ALS.

changes, and constipation. Any or all of these problems can cause your caloric and nutrient intake to decline, resulting in weight loss. You may lose some body fat with unplanned weight loss, but you can also lose muscle mass. This will weaken you and can adversely affect your immune status. Moreover, ALS is a *hypermetabolic* disease: one that causes you to use more calories and nutrients than normal.

Therefore, you need extra calories to maintain yourself during this period. A healthy diet helps provide a sense of well-being, maintains your immune status, and keeps you in a desirable weight range. It is vital to maintain good health by eating right!

What Can the Dietitian Do to Help?

The primary role of the dietitian is to help you improve your quality of life through healthy eating habits. The dietitian will ask you questions about your meal pattern, the foods that you eat, and in what amounts you eat them. The nutritional assessment will be made after taking into consideration factors that include your age, height, weight, activity pattern, and the progression of your disease. This assessment is a comprehensive evaluation of your nutritional needs and recommendations to help you succeed. The dietitian will monitor your progress, provide ongoing support, and help you build your capacity for achieving optimal health.

The dietitian may ask you questions that relate to your nutritional status—for example: "How is your appetite? Has your weight changed recently?" Monitoring your weight is one way to see how well you are doing. Your weight will be stable if you continue to eat regularly and your activity remains the same. As mentioned above, some patients with ALS will lose weight. You may be asking yourself, "How can I be using more calories when I am less active?" Think about when you have the flu. Your body becomes hypermetabolic: it works harder to combat the illness, expends more calories, and often loses weight. This becomes a health concern if symptoms do not resolve quickly.

The dietitian often works with a speech therapist if you have swallowing difficulties. They are both good resources for addressing nutritional concerns, promoting healthy eating, and reducing the incidence of complications.

Ensuring Good Nutrition

One way to ensure you have good nutrition is to plan your meals and snacks using the *Food Guide Pyramid* (Figure 7-1). You may recognize it as the evolved version of what we commonly call the "Four Basic Food Groups: Milk, Meat, Fruits and Vegetables, and Breads and Cereals." Building your diet based on these guidelines is a good way of making sure you maintain optimal nutrition.

> One way to ensure you have good nutrition is to plan your meals and snacks using the *Food Guide Pyramid*.

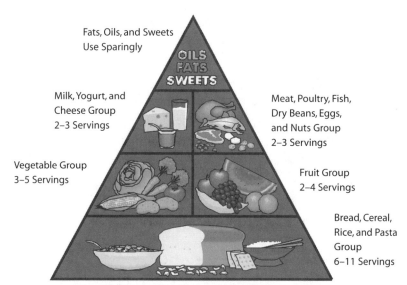

Fats, Oils, and Sweets
Use Sparingly

Milk, Yogurt, and
Cheese Group
2–3 Servings

Meat, Poultry, Fish,
Dry Beans, Eggs,
and Nuts Group
2–3 Servings

Vegetable Group
3–5 Servings

Fruit Group
2–4 Servings

Bread, Cereal,
Rice, and Pasta
Group
6–11 Servings

Select a section of the pyramid for details

The Food Guide Pyramid is an outline of what to eat each day based on the Dietary Guidelines. It's not a rigid prescription but a general guide that lets you choose a healthful diet that's right for you.

The Pyramid calls for eating a variety of foods to get the nutrients you need and at the same time the right amount of calories to maintain healthy weight.

Use the Pyramid to help you eat better every day…the Dietary Guidelines way. Start with plenty of breads, cereals, rice, pasta, vegetables, and fruits. Add 2–3 servings from the milk group and 2–3 servings from the meat group. Remember to go easy on fats, oils, and sweets, the foods in the small tip of the Pyramid.

What Counts as One Serving?

The amount of food that counts as one serving is listed below. If you eat a larger portion, count it as more than 1 serving. For example, a dinner portion of spaghetti would count as 2 or 3 servings of pasta.

Be sure to eat at least the lowest number of servings from the five major food groups listed below. You need them for the vitamins, minerals, carbohydrates, and protein they provide. Just try to pick the lowest fat choices from the food groups. No specific serving size is given for the fats, oils, and sweets group because the message is USE SPARINGLY.

Milk, Yogurt, and Cheese

1 cup of milk or yogurt	1 1/2 ounces of natural cheese	2 ounces of process cheese

Meat, Poultry, Fish, Dry Beans, Eggs, and Nuts

2-3 ounces of cooked lean meat, poultry, or fish
1/2 cup of cooked dry beans, 1 egg, or 2 tablespoons of peanut butter count as 1 ounce of lean meat

Vegetables

1 cup of raw leafy vegetables	1/2 cup of other vegetables, cooked or chopped raw	3/4 cup of vegetable juice

Fruit

1 medium apple, banana, orange	1/2 cup of chopped, cooked, or canned fruit	3/4 cup of fruit juice

Bread, Cereal, Rice, and Pasta

1 slice of bread	1 ounce of ready-to-eat cereal	1/2 cup of cooked cereal, rice, or pasta

FIGURE 7-1

The food guide pyramid: A guide to daily food choices.

The Food Guide Pyramid is an outline of what to eat each day based on the Dietary Guidelines. It is not a rigid prescription but a general guide that lets you choose a healthful diet that is right for you. (Go to this Web site for more details: http://www.nal.usda.gov/fnic/Fpyr/pmap.htm.)

The Food Guide Pyramid suggests how many servings you should have daily and examples of serving sizes are given. Make sure you eat at least the lowest number of servings daily from each food group. Also, keep in mind that eating a variety from each of the four food groups provides the nutrients you need and at the same time the right amount of calories to help maintain a healthy weight. The tip of the pyramid has fats, oils, and sweets. You should use less of these foods if you are watching your weight. For those people who may need to *gain* weight, fats, oils, and sweets can help add calories without adding volume to meals.

One way to see if you are eating right is to keep a food diary. Write down everything you eat. At the end of 3 days, check to see how many servings you consumed from each food group. Then you can make the appropriate changes in your diet.

Adding Protein to Maintain Muscle

Protein is found in meat, fish, poultry, milk, cheese, eggs, beans, and legumes. They are the building blocks of muscle. Try to get the suggested 2 to 3 servings per day. Some people with ALS have difficulty consuming enough protein, usually because they experience difficulty with chewing and swallowing meats. Mealtimes may be longer due to fatigue in chewing. Here are some ways to increase protein in your diet:

- Add grated cheese to vegetables, soups, and salads.
- Use milk instead of water in making hot chocolate.
- Add instant breakfast mixes to a glass of milk.
- Add tofu to sauces, soups, or meat loaf.
- Use cottage cheese on a baked potato.
- Add a can of cannelloni beans to a casserole or sauce.
- Add nonfat dry milk powder to cream soups, casseroles, sauces, and gravies.
- Chop up hardboiled eggs to top off casseroles, soups, and creamed vegetable dishes.

TABLE 7-1

Food Groups—Example of One Serving.

Breads, Grains, and Cereals 6-11 servings:	Meat Group 2-3 servings:
1 slice of bread	1/2 cup cottage cheese, tuna fish,
1/2 bagel	chicken salad
1/2 cup of mashed potatoes, rice, or pasta	4 tbl. peanut butter
1 small baked potato	2–3 ounces of meat, fish, poultry
1/2 cup cooked cereal	(the size of a deck of cards)
3/4 cup dry cereal	1/2 cup soy bean curd (tofu)
one 7" tortilla	1/2 cup cooked dry beans

Fruit Group 2-4 servings:	Vegetable Group 3-5 servings:
1 piece of fresh fruit	1/2 cup cooked vegetables
1/2 cup canned fruit	1 cup of raw vegetables
1/2 cup fruit juice	

Milk Group 2-3 servings:
1 cup of milk or yogurt
1 1/2 ounces of natural cheese
2 ounces of processed cheese

Adding Calories to Maintain Weight

Your body begins to break down muscle for energy when you do not take in enough calories. Foods high in fat and sugar are concentrated sources of calories. You can add fats, such as butter, margarine, oil, and salad dressings, to improve the taste and smoothness of your meals. Here are some tips:

- Add an extra pat of butter, margarine, or oil to soups, baked chicken, fish, pasta, potatoes, rice, casseroles, gravies, or sauces.
- Add an extra tablespoon of mayonnaise, butter, or margarine to your bread when making sandwiches. You could also add more mayonnaise to egg salad, tuna fish, and chicken salad.
- Add sugar, honey, jam, or jelly to sweeten hot or cold cereals, yogurt, or ice cream.
- Use ice cream in making milkshakes, smoothies, or floats.

Vitamin and Mineral Supplements

You may have questions about what kinds of vitamin and mineral supplements you should take, and your doctor may recommend certain vitamins and minerals for you. In particular, supplementation of antioxidants (such as vitamin E) may be of benefit.

Vitamin E is a *fat soluble* vitamin. Alpha tocopherol is the most powerful antioxidant of the eight different forms of vitamin E. Antioxidants prevent cellular damage by free radicals. Free radicals are destructive molecules that are by-products of cell metabolism. Their interaction with other molecules causes cellular damage. Vitamin E is an antioxidant that stabilizes free radicals and prevents neurotoxic effects.

Food sources of vitamin E include vegetable oils, (olive, sunflower, safflower, cottonseed, and soy oils), wheat germ, avocados, nuts, and whole grain products. It is recommended that adults 19 years and older receive 15 International Units (I.U.) (1 mg alpha tocopherol = 1.5 International Units).

Your doctor may recommend vitamin E supplements to help fight ALS. The daily dosage may range from 400 to 2,000 I.U.

Vitamin E should *only* be taken under the guidance of your physician, especially if you are also taking anticoagulants or blood thinners (such as Coumadin®). High doses of vitamin E may cause gastrointestinal upset.

Other antioxidants, include vitamin C, alpha-lipoic acid, and n-acetylcysteine; however, no studies have shown benefit from these. Any other nutritional supplements you are taking should be discussed with your doctor because they may or may not be beneficial.

Managing Nutritional Concerns

Recommended Body Weight

Plan to maintain your usual weight. Occasionally people with ALS will notice that their clothes are feeling tight or that they need to go to a larger waist size. This may be the result of a loss of muscle tone in the abdominal area. Avoid trying to lose weight by dieting. It is not uncommon for patients with ALS to lose some weight due to losing muscle mass. If you feel you are overweight, do not diet to lose weight, because it may become more difficult to eat later on. The dietitian can work with you to meet your

> **Plan to maintain your usual weight.**

nutritional needs, achieve a balanced diet, and maintain your weight. By telling the dietitian what foods and how much you eat, she can make suggestions to modify your daily intake while still achieving a balanced diet.

Will ALS Affect My Appetite?

The voluntary muscles that are involved in eating may weaken because of ALS, causing changes in how much you eat and what foods you can eat. You may experience problems with chewing and swallowing. It may be difficult for you to prepare your own food and to feed yourself. You may have problems with constipation, become easily fatigued, and have a depressed appetite. Any or all of these can result in undesired weight loss and cause you to feel weaker. It is important to discuss these changes in your appetite and ability to eat with the doctor and the dietitian. There are ways to address these nutritional concerns.

Chewing and Swallowing Difficulties

Consult a speech therapist, who can assess your ability to chew and swallow, or a dietitian for suggestions if you have problems keeping up with your nutritional needs. Changing the texture of your foods may help you chew and swallow more easily. Soft foods with higher moisture content, such as meat loaf, casseroles, chicken salad, egg salad, and tuna fish, are usually easier to swallow.

Liquids can be thickened to ease swallowing. The dietitian may recommend some commercial products that can be added to foods and liquids to achieve the recommended consistency (Table 7-2). Recipe books are also available with easy-to-prepare and easy-to-eat foods.

TABLE 7-2

Food Products—Commercial Thickeners

Thicken-Up™	Nutra-thick™ (Menu Magic)
Thickit™	Classic Instant Food Thickener™

There may be times when you have little appetite or energy to eat. A dietitian may recommend that you add nutritional supplements such as Ensure™ or Boost™ to your meal plan. These supplements will provide you with essential protein, fat, carbohydrates, vitamins, and minerals in the form of liquid nutrition. Use these supplements as a meal or take them as part of your meal.

Swallowing Tips

You may experience difficulty swallowing foods and liquids. The first sign may be coughing when swallowing water. With swallowing difficulties, you may tire easily when chewing, have problems moving food with your tongue, and have food get stuck in your throat. If you experience any of these symptoms, request a swallowing evaluation. A speech therapist may be able to teach you swallowing techniques and recommend what food consistency is best and safest for you.

The following are some ideas to make swallowing easier:

Environment and Atmosphere While Eating
- Eat in quiet and pleasant surroundings. Avoid the television and radio, which may distract you from eating.
- Positioning: Sit up straight in a firm chair with your head slightly forward and your chin down, or follow the specific positioning recommended by your doctor or speech therapist.
- Avoid eating alone. You may feel safer eating your meals with someone. Ask the clinic staff to teach family members the Heimlich maneuver.
- Use seasonings and sauces and smell your foods. This will help stimulate your appetite and salivary glands.

- Do not talk while eating. Swallow your food before talking.
- Complete swallowing before breathing again.
- Take one small bite at a time. Eat slowly, taking small bites and chew your food well.
- Try sipping from a straw. This helps to keep chin tucked and sip sizes smaller.
- Alternate between eating and drinking. Take a bite of food and then sip some liquid.
- Cough when you need to, as it will prevent food from going down your airway.
- When you cough, swallow immediately before taking a breath.
- After eating, sit upright for at least 20 minutes. This will aid in digestion and also help in preventing heartburn.

Modifying Food Texture or Consistency
- Try cold, flavorful, or carbonated liquids if you are beginning to experience problems with thin liquids. These provide stimulation in the mouth that can trigger a swallow.
- Drinking thicker liquids such as nectars, milkshakes, and smoothies will be better tolerated than thin liquids. (Thick liquids move more slowly down your throat instead of spreading out the way thin liquids do. Also, thick liquids are less likely go down your airway.)
- Thicken fruit juices with pureed fruit.
- Blend puddings or custards into milk to thicken them.
- Soft and smooth foods are easier to chew and swallow. These foods are higher in moisture (e.g., meat loaf vs. a steak). Use extra sauces and gravies to moisten your foods.
- Foods with one texture or a single consistency will be easier to swallow. A thick cream soup is easier to swallow than a minestrone or meat and vegetable soup.

Commercial thickeners: You could use any of the products noted in Table 7-2 to mix liquids to the recommended consistency.

Foods that may be difficult to swallow are listed in Table 7-3.

TABLE 7-3

Foods to Avoid Because of Difficulty Swallowing

- Extra-spicy, "hot," or acidic foods
- Soft fresh bread
- Cookies, crackers, dry cereal, and graham crackers
- Dry muffins and cake
- Dry, fibrous, or bony meats and fish
- Coconut and pineapple
- Sticky foods (for example: peanut butter)
- Stringy vegetables (for example: lettuce and celery)
- Fried noodles and rice
- Popcorn, potato chips, and nuts
- Fruits and vegetables with skin or seeds (for example: peas, corn, apples, and berries)

A 57-year-old man with ALS lost 20 pounds from his baseline weight. He complained of fatigue with chewing. The unplanned weight loss contributed to his weakness and lethargy. It was suggested that he switch to a mechanical soft diet that included foods that were soft-textured, moist, and easier to swallow. The dietitian recommended that meats be moistened and ground-up or minced; foods to include in his diet were casseroles, meat, salads, and soups. He was cautioned to avoid dry, coarse foods, such as seeds, nuts, raw vegetables, and fruits. Also he was encouraged to eat six small meals per day. His in-between snacks consisted of liquid nutritional supplements. His appetite improved and his weight stabilized.

Comment: *Suggestions to change the texture of his foods greatly enhanced his caloric intake. These changes also helped stop further undesirable weight loss.*

Fatigue

Consider having six small meals each day if it is difficult for you to eat three large meals. Your in-between meals or snacks can be nutritional supplements recommended by the dietitian.

Constipation

You may experience problems with constipation. Constipation can result from a number of things. It may be harder for you to drink enough fluids, eat enough fiber, and get enough exercise. Some medications can lead to constipation. In addition, with ALS your abdominal muscles weaken, which contributes to the inability to bear down in moving your bowels. Whatever the reason, constipation is very uncomfortable and will depress your appetite. The following suggestions may help you avoid this problem.

Increase fluids. Consume at least eight cups of fluid daily. Caffeine and alcoholic beverages cause dehydration and should not be considered as part of your eight cups of daily fluids. Drinking plenty of liquids will

> Consume at least eight cups of fluid daily.

help prevent dehydration and constipation. Signs of dehydration include dry mouth, dark-colored urine, and sudden weight loss. Contact your doctor or nurse immediately if you experience any of these symptoms.

Increase fiber. Taking in a good amount of fiber will also help you avoid constipation. Fiber is carbohydrate that cannot be digested. All plant foods have fiber, including fruits, vegetables, legumes, and grains. There are basically two different kinds of fiber: soluble fiber that partially dissolves in water and insoluble fiber that does not dissolve in water (Table 7-4).

Both types of fiber play a part in reducing the risk of certain diseases, such as heart disease, diverticular disease, and type 2 diabetes. It is recom-

TABLE 7-4
Soluble and Insoluble Fiber

Soluble Fiber	Insoluble Fiber
oatmeal, oat bran nuts and seeds apples, strawberries, blueberries carrots, cucumbers, pears, zucchini, celery, tomatoes, and whole dried peas	whole-grain breakfast cereals wheat bran, seeds grains found in whole wheat breads, barley, beans and lentils, couscous, brown rice and bulgur

mended you get at least 20 to 35 grams of fiber each day. If you do not have problems swallowing, plan to include eight servings daily of high fiber foods. (Follow the Food Guide Pyramid recommendations for serving sizes, Figure 7-1.) If you have problems swallowing, you may need to avoid eating dry, coarse products, such as whole grain breads and cereals, which contain nuts and seeds. Instead, consume more fruits and vegetables to increase fiber. Eat canned fruits and vegetables for softer texture.

Prunes and prune juice can also help regulate your bowels. (See Table 7-5 for suggested recipes.) There are also some "Anti-Constipation" recipes on the Lou Gehrig Disease Web site you might like to try (http://www.lougehrigsdisease.net).

TABLE 7-5

Recipes for Constipation

Prune Juice Cocktail

*1/2 cup applesauce
2 tablespoonfuls miller's bran
4-6 ounces prune juice

Take 1 tablespoonful per day (increase as needed).

*The amount of applesauce can be 4-ounce package.

Anticonstipation Fruit Paste

1 pound prunes
1 pound raisins
1 pound figs
1 cup lemon juice
1 cup brown sugar
*4-ounce package Senna tea

Steep tea 5 minutes in 3-1/2 cups of boiling water. Strain. Add fruit to 2 cups of tea and boil for 5 minutes. Add sugar and lemon juice. Cool. Use food processor or blender to turn mixture into a smooth paste. Put in a plastic container and place in freezer.

Take 1 or 2 tablespoonfuls daily.

*Senna tea adjusted to personal taste. You may wish to start with 1/8 cup and add over time.

Nutritional Supplements with Fiber Stool Softeners or Bulk Laxatives

(Talk to your doctor about any other recommendations.)

Ensure™ with Fiber, Colace™, Boost™ with fiber, Metamucil™, Nutren™ with Fiber.

Summary

There are two ways you can monitor whether you are meeting your nutritional needs. First, make sure you are following the guidelines in the Food Guide Pyramid. Second, weigh yourself once a week and keep a record of your weight. It is a good idea to weigh in at the same time on the same day wearing similar clothing (or no clothing) every week. Tell your doctor and dietitian if you notice your weight is dropping.

Despite the challenges you may face in consuming enough nourishment to meet your nutritional needs, your doctor and dietitian can work with you to address them. It is important that you communicate your questions and concerns so they can be proactive in helping you maintain optimal nutritional health.

When You Can't Keep Up with Your Nutritional Needs

There is good news even if you are still losing weight, despite changing the types and consistency of foods that you eat and adding calories and protein by drinking commercially available liquid supplements. If you are unable to keep up with your caloric needs by mouth, you can meet all or some of your nutritional needs by using the liquid supplements in a different way. A feeding tube can be placed directly into your stomach that will completely bypass problematic chewing and swallowing. However, this feeding tube will not prevent you from continuing to eat the foods you enjoy by mouth. Continuing to eat and drink while also supplementing by tube works well for many people with ALS.

A percutaneous endoscopic gastrostomy (PEG) tube can be placed by a gastroenterologist: a physician who specializes in the treatment of diseases of the gastrointestinal tract. The procedure for placing the tube is relatively simple. The back of the throat is numbed; a sedative is given intravenously that relaxes you (but you remain awake during the procedure); a tube, about the diameter of a drinking straw, is advanced down the throat and guided by an instrument (endoscope) that allows the physician to visualize the esophagus, the muscular passage that runs from the throat to the stomach, and the stomach. The skin over the stomach area is numbed with a local anesthetic and a small incision is made; the feeding tube is threaded down the endoscope into the stomach and pulled through the incision. The feeding tube stays in place by positioning a small balloon against the stomach wall internally and another balloon externally against the skin of the abdomen. Oxygen levels, blood pressure, and heart rate are monitored during the procedure, which takes about 20 minutes. Most people find that they remember nothing about the procedure because of the sedative that is used. You will have some discomfort for a few days, but you can resume normal activities and can begin showering or swimming shortly thereafter. You can begin feedings through your new PEG tube the day after it is placed.

The procedure is safest and easiest while the breathing capacity is strong (50 percent of predicted or above) and before a person becomes malnourished. Ideally, you will have a feeding tube placed while you are still able to eat. The feeding tube will not affect your ability to swallow. Often you can continue eating but will use the tube for water, taking pills, and also some liquid food supplement each day. The only maintenance needed is flushing the tube daily with water so it does not get clogged. Pouring the supplement into the tube is quite easy; it works by gravity and is similar to putting oil into your car. A dietitian will recommend the type and amount of liquid supplement needed to fulfill your nutritional requirements. If needed, all of your nutritional needs can be met with liquid supplementation. You might consider the feeding tube as an insurance policy to be used when you need it.

Linda came to ALS clinic with predominantly bulbar symptoms of speech and swallowing difficulty. She had lost 20 pounds over the course of a year, was finding that meals took an hour to eat, and was using high-calorie additions to her meals yet continuing to lose weight. She was tired and constipated much of the time. Her husband Jim was constantly nagging her to eat more and was frightened by her continued weight loss. At the clinic visit, her pulmonary function test was 60 percent of predicted. She broke down and cried when a PEG tube was recommended by her doctor saying, "I won't feel attractive with a tube sticking out of me. How can I go out to dinner with my friends if I cannot eat anymore?"

Linda was surprised when she saw how flexible the tube was and that it could not be seen through her clothing. Her husband was able to tell her that he hated nagging her but was really worried about her weight loss. They talked with the gastroenterologist and decided to have the procedure after the holidays. Linda stayed in the hospital overnight and the nutritionist instructed her in how to do her feedings. She was discharged knowing how to independently care for her feeding tube and with a prescription for a pain medicine that she used for 2 days. One month later, she had gained 3 pounds, had more energy, and was having regular bowel movements. She found that she could take her supplements before going out to dinner with friends and then eat a small amount, just for the pleasure of tasting food without worrying about eating enough. She no longer choked on her pills and water because she used her tube for these things. Her relationship with her husband was much improved. Her comment to the doctor was, "I don't know why I waited so long."

Comment: *The decision to have a feeding tube is a major one. Fears of being unattractive and dependent on medical interventions are common. Conflict with loved ones about weight loss can be intense. The insertion of a feeding tube can simplify and prolong life, improve energy, reduce conflict, and produce a general sense of well-being.*

CHAPTER 8

Speech, Communication, and Computer Access

Amy Roman, MS, CCC-SLP

Maintaining the ability to communicate is essential for everyone diagnosed with ALS. In this chapter, we will discuss the changes you may experience that affect communication and explain why they occur. These

> Maintaining the ability to communicate is essential.

changes may be in speech or they may be in hand function for writing and keyboarding. Both are important for communication and will be addressed. We will also explain the steps you can take to ensure your ability to communicate effectively throughout the course of your illness.

After being diagnosed, you may be concerned because you already notice some changes in your speech. Perhaps you have not experienced any problems but have heard that many people with ALS eventually have difficulty talking. It should be quite reassuring, therefore, to learn that although speech changes do occur in most patients with ALS, communication with loved ones, care providers, and your community can be maintained by working closely with a qualified speech language pathologist. As always, knowledge is your most powerful tool and there is much to be learned. The biggest challenge for many patients with ALS is getting past their fears and preparing themselves with education and action. Your speech language pathologist will be your partner in this effort.

The wife of a 43-year-old man with ALS attended a support group meeting on speech and communication with ALS. She reported that her husband refused to come to the lecture; he said, "When I can no longer surf and no longer speak, I do not want to live anymore." Two years later, this patient co-presented the lecture on communication from his wheelchair alongside the speech language pathologist. He was completely nonspeaking by this point and gave his part of the presentation using a communication device. He had preprogrammed the device to "speak" his part of the lecture and he also composed on-the-spot jokes and responses to questions from the audience.

Comment: *This patient's initial reaction is common, as is his gradual transition into acceptance. This transition often involves serious philosophical reflection. With time and thought, he was able to adjust his priorities, take a strong leadership role in the management of his own communication, and become an important mentor to others.*

Normal Speech

To understand why speech problems occur, we need a basic understanding of the speech process. Producing speech involves a complex series of events that happen in a coordinated way. All speech sounds begin as air in the lungs. The force with which air is expelled from the lungs controls the volume of speech. The exhaled air is silent until it passes through the vocal

> Producing speech involves a complex series of events that happen in a coordinated way.

cords. The vocal cords create sound in much the same way as the strings of a guitar do when strummed. The vocal cords begin to vibrate when air passes though them as it leaves the lungs. This vibration creates a tone. The tone is then directed into either the mouth or the nose by the *soft palate*, the back part of the roof of the mouth. Usually, the soft palate lifts to block the nasal passage when we speak so that air is directed through the mouth. The tone is then further modified by the tongue, lips, and jaw. All three must form extremely precise, synchronized movements to create each distinct sound of the alphabet. These sounds, which are produced rapidly and in a specific order, create the words we say.

How Does ALS Affect Speech?

Dysarthria is the name of the speech disorder associated with ALS. Typically, speech becomes increasingly slurred, slow, and nasal. There may also be changes in the pitch and volume of the voice. These changes are due to the loss of nerve connections to the muscles that move the lungs, vocal cords, lips, tongue, jaw, and soft palate. This loss causes weakness, stiffness, and reduced coordination in these essential speech muscles.

Reduced muscle function has an effect on each part of the speech anatomy. The lungs are the "power house" of speech. ALS weakens the diaphragm and other muscles that allow us to breathe properly. Patients find that their voice becomes softer and difficult to hear without adequate breath support. They may also notice that they cannot produce as many words per breath as they once could. Often whole words or the ends of words are lost because the speaker reaches the end of a breath before the words are completely expressed.

As explained above, air from the lungs moves through the vocal cords to produce sound. When the muscles of the vocal cords are weakened or tightened by ALS, the pitch of your voice may be higher, lower, or change suddenly. This is similar to the way the pitch of a guitar changes when you tighten or loosen the strings.

Next, the soft palate directs the tone, either through the nose or the mouth. In the English language, most speech sounds are produced through the mouth, "m" and "n" being the exceptions. Many people with ALS find that all of their sounds pass through their nose. This occurs because the weakened soft palate is unable to lift during speech to block air from passing though the nose. As a result of this open nasal airflow, speech sounds become distorted. For example, when spoken by someone with nasal speech, the letters "p" and "b" sound similar to "m." Thus, the words "pie" and "bye" sound instead like "my."

Loss of range of movement and strength in the tongue, lips, and jaw often cause the first noticeable signs of dysarthria. This occurs because the timing and precision of their movements must be exact to form recognizable speech sounds. Notice all of the changes in the position of your tongue, lips, and jaw when, for example, you say the word "parakeet." Now try to lock your jaw, tongue, and lips in one position and say the same word. This gives you an idea of the slurring effect caused by having reduced function in these muscles. This diminished muscle function also may cause speech to be slower than normal. Patients say that they just cannot form the words as quickly as they think of them.

All of these factors, alone or in combination, can make it very difficult for listeners to understand the speech of people with ALS. Initially, a

> A speech language pathologist may provide suggestions to improve speech intelligibility and reduce communication breakdowns.

speech language pathologist may provide suggestions to improve speech intelligibility and reduce communication breakdowns. Some popular and simple strategies to improve communication include the following:

- Provide listeners with the topic you are going to talk about. This makes it easier for a listener to fill in the gaps if some of your words are unclear.
- Speak slowly and concentrate on including each sound in words. Focus especially on the sound at the end of each word that is frequently dropped (e.g., cat, talk, jar).
- Exaggerate your lip, tongue, and jaw movements to make words sound clear.
- Take deep breaths more frequently, even in the middle of sentences. Your first few words after a breath will be the clearest.
- Be aware of your environment and avoid having conversations in noisy areas.

- Be aware of your energy level. The speech of many people with ALS becomes less clear as the day progresses. Plan important conversations or phone calls for your peak energy times.
- Gain your listener's attention before you begin speaking. The listener's ability to understand your words will be improved if they are focused on you and able to look at your face while you speak.
- Teach your listeners how to help. You may ask a listener to give you a signal to remind you to slow down and speak clearly instead of interrupting with "I do not understand." You may also suggest that listeners repeat what they did understand, so you will know exactly what part of the sentence you need to repeat when there is a communication breakdown.

What You Can Do at Various Stages

Stage One: What to Do Before Any Speech Changes Occur

It is never too early to prepare yourself in a few simple ways in case your speech becomes difficult to understand. If you have been thinking about

> It is never too early to prepare yourself in a few simple ways in case your speech becomes difficult to understand.

learning to use a computer, the Internet, or e-mail, now is the time. Computers provide an excellent means of communication, both for people with limited mobility and those with speech difficulties.

A 68-year-old patient with severe speech difficulties found that she relied more and more on e-mail for communication. She noted that she felt on par with others because timing was not an issue as it is in phone communication. No one was waiting for her to produce messages and she felt no pressure to abridge her thoughts. She even stated that when writing and reading e-mails, she could almost forget she had ALS.

Now is also a good time to begin *voice banking*—recording messages, greetings, requests, expressions, stories, jokes, or anything else that you say frequently. These recordings of your own voice can later be used in an augmentative-alternative communication (AAC) device or to preserve stories for your family and friends. Ask your speech language pathologist for instructions on recording directly into your computer. The sound recording program that allows you to record and save your voice in the form of wav.files is already in most computers under "Accessories." You can easily organize your recordings by giving each file a useful name (e.g., "familiar greeting," "formal greeting," "leaving phone message," "story about Ted," etc.). Ask your speech language pathologist or ALSA/MDA chapter for a list of common messages you can record.

Stage Two: What to Do When Detectable Speech Changes Begin

You should make an appointment with a speech language pathologist at the first sign of any change in your speech. You need to find a speech language pathologist who has worked with patients with ALS or who is an

> Make an appointment with a speech language pathologist at the first sign of any change in your speech.

augmentative-alternative communication specialist, preferably both. Referrals may be available through your local or national ALS Association, Muscular Dystrophy Association, your neurologist, the local university, or the American Speech and Hearing Association. Contact information is included in the Resources section at the end of this chapter.

Your speech language pathologist will begin monitoring your speech changes and provide you with education and communication strategies as needed. It is important for him to get a baseline measurement of the rate at which you speak and your intelligibility. You may be asked to read a short passage to provide these measurements. He will examine your mouth and breathing, and assess your voice quality. He will also evaluate your hand functioning for writing and keyboard use. Your speech language pathologist may suggest some gentle oral stretches or massage techniques to relax tight muscles. Oral strengthening exercises are not recommended because they are not effective in improving the speech muscles.

A small hands-free voice amplifier may be appropriate if your speech is difficult for others to hear or if you have to strain to project your voice. You also may want to set up an alert system at home if your voice is not strong enough to call out for assistance. Wireless door chimes or infant monitors work well. If you have difficulty pressing a chime button, EnablingDevices.com offers adapted attendant call chimes and personal pagers. These chimes or pagers are adapted to be activated with a switch.

You may want to ask your speech language pathologist if a *palatal lift* might be helpful if your voice is nasal. This is a prosthetic device that lifts your soft palate and reduces the escape of air through the nose.

You may also want to look into the telephone access program in your state. Being understood over the phone is particularly challenging for many people with ALS. Most states offer free services that assist people with speech and mobility and manipulation disabilities to continue to use the phone.

Stage Three: What to Do When Speech Begins to Become Difficult to Understand

Ask your speech language pathologist to provide you with strategies to improve intelligibility and to help avoid or repair communication breakdowns.

Initial letter cuing is an additional strategy that is remarkably effective in improving intelligibility when patients are having regular communication breakdowns. It is a simple procedure but it does take some practice. As the patient speaks, he points to the first letter of each of his words on an ABC board (see Figure 8-1A). This strategy provides the listener with information

FIGURE 8-1A

Simple ABC board.

Space A B C D E F G H

I J K L M N O P Q R S

T U V W X Y Z   Delete

1 2 3 4 5 6 7 8 9 0 Ask me yes/no questions

Say and write down each letter as I point to it.

about the first sound in each word and also where each word begins and ends. Additionally, it helps the person with ALS learn to speak more slowly, thereby producing all of the sounds in each word more efficiently. Many people utilize this strategy mainly when they have had a communication breakdown and verbal repetitions of the sentence have not been helpful.

Even if you are only occasionally having communication breakdowns, it may be time for you and your speech language pathologist to begin the process of obtaining a high-tech AAC device. Speech generating devices are covered by Medicare and most private insurance. Unfortunately, the time between scheduling the AAC evaluation, obtaining insurance approval, and finally receiving the device can be many months. Beginning this process early will allow you to become skilled in using your device and customize it thoroughly before you actually need to use it as your primary mode of communication.

Stage 4: What to Do When Speech Is Not Functional for Communication

At this stage, you will most likely be using a low-tech or possibly a high-tech AAC system. Successful users of this technology have a number of things in common. Possibly the most important is that they continue to work closely with their speech language pathologist. You and your speech language pathologist should develop different strategies to use depending on your fatigue level, your location, and the person with whom you are communicating. Many of the most successful AAC users implement a variety of communication strategies throughout their day.

FIGURE 8-1B

ABC and core vocabulary board.

How	What	A	B	C	D	E	F	G	H	I	J	please	thanks	day	now	time
When	Where	K	L	M	N	O	P	Qu	R	S	Delete	Bad	Good	Today	Tomorrow	Yesterday
Who	Why	Yes	T	U	V	W	X	Y	Z	No	?	Cold	Hot	Bag	Bathroom	bed
I	Me	My	To	Be	Call	change	Come	A	Any	Every	Some	More	Much	Car	Chair	medicine
It	We	Am	Are	Drink	Eat	Feel	Find	All	About	And	At	Okay	Tired	Pain	Pillow	TV
He	Him	Can	Could	Get	Give	Go	Help	That	Because	But	by	Really	Very	1	2	3
She	Her	Did	Do	Hurt	Know	Like	Love	The	Down	For	From	Forward	Back	4	5	6
They	Their	Had	Has	Make	Move	Need	Put	This	Here	If	In	Left	Right	7	8	9
You	Your	Have	Is	Rub	Say	Scratch	Take	-ed	Of	Off	On	Sunday	Uncomfortable	$	0	:
Don't	Not	Was	Were	Talk	Tell	Think	Use	-ing	Or	Out	Over	Monday	Tuesday	Wed.	:00	:15
Can't	Won't	Will	Would	Walk	Want	Watch	Work	-s	There	Up	With	Thurs.	Fri.	Sat.	:30	:45

WordPower™ by Nancy Inman (Available through Saltillo Corp. www.saltillo.com)

A 56-year-old man with ALS begins his day using speech to communicate with his wife; they have developed strategies to resolve communication breakdowns. He repeats words frequently and, if she is still unable to understand, he uses gestures or spells the word aloud. An attendant arrives to assist him while his wife is at work. English is not her first language and she is not able to understand his speech. He mainly uses a low-tech communication book with the attendant that contains his most common requests. Occasionally, when he has an unanticipated request for her, he points to letters on an ABC board to spell out his message, although this is fatiguing for him. During the day, he uses his computer (which is also a speech generating device) to e-mail friends and post messages to different user groups. He also preprograms messages in the device in preparation for anticipated conversations or appointments. He does not use a regular keyboard because he has arm weakness. He uses a joystick to select letters on a keyboard that is displayed on his computer screen and relies heavily on rate enhancement features like word prediction. By dinner time, his energy is low and speaking is impossible. He now uses his AAC device to "speak" messages he preprogrammed during the day to, for example, ask his daughter about her S.A.T. preparation and tell a funny story about the attendant. When his wife mentions car troubles, he is able to have an impromptu conversation with her about car maintenance during which he uses rate enhancement features to speed up his communication.

It is essential to work with your speech language pathologist as your physical abilities change in order to make the necessary adjustments to your system. All systems require routine modifications to keep them as effortless as possible.

What Is Augmentative-Alternate Communication or "AAC"?

Augmentative-alternative communication is any method of communication that supplements or replaces speech for people with severe speech impairments. As speech becomes somewhat difficult for others to under-

> Augmentative-alternative communication is any method of communication that supplements or replaces speech for people with severe speech impairments.

stand, people with ALS often use various methods to augment or enhance their own speech. One method of AAC that is popular with ALS patients is *voice amplification.*

A 76-year-old patient had difficulty being understood by her husband, who has a mild hearing loss. Friends were also having problems understanding her in public places, such as restaurants. Her breathing strength was reduced and her speech was soft, although her speech was only mildly slurred and still easy to understand. The problem was solved with four simple solutions. She borrowed a small hands-free voice amplifier from her ALS Association's lending library. She also borrowed a wireless door chime that allowed her to call her husband when he was in another room. She and her friends also found quieter restaurants where they could meet. Additionally, her husband was fitted for hearing aids.

Comment: *By augmenting her speech and enlisting the help of her friends in finding practical solutions, this patient was able to maintain and possibly prolong her ability to speak as well as conserve energy. AAC equipment is often available through lending libraries run by clinics, ALSA, and MDA chapters.*

As important as it is to try to maintain the effective use of your own speech through methods that augment it, it is also important to recognize when your speech has become impossible for others to understand. Many patients have difficulty accepting this transition. Friends and care providers need to be sensitive, honest, and direct if your speech has become impossible for them to understand.

Your speech language pathologist will help you to develop alternative methods for communication. Hundreds of AAC systems are available, so it is essential that a knowledgeable speech language pathologist customizes the solutions that best match your needs and abilities. Both low-tech and high-tech AAC options should be explored because each has advantages.

Low-Tech Augmentative-Alternative Communication

Augmentative-alternative communication methods that do not require electricity or that use very simple or no equipment are referred to as "low-technology" or "no-technology." Often these systems can be created using material you have in your home. Examples of low-tech/no-tech AAC include:

- Writing messages on a pad of paper or a reusable writing board.
- Pointing to letters, words, or messages on communication boards.
- Using facial expressions, gestures, or sign language.
- Using a sound or gesture to indicate your choice when presented with a series of options (examples of gestures include: eye glance up/down, left/right, eye blinks, raised finger, raised eyebrow, specific head movement, etc.).
- Using gestures to indicate "yes" and "no" when provided with a series of yes/no questions that begin broadly and become more specific.
- Using an alerting or call system, such as a bell, wireless door chime, or infant monitor.

Communication boards are a popular and simple low-tech way to communicate when handwriting becomes slow, illegible, or fatiguing. The board is usually made of paper, cardboard, or Plexiglas, and the patient composes messages by selecting letters, words, or phrases presented on the board. The person who is communicating with the patient (the communication partner) often repeats aloud each selection so that the patient knows

> Communication boards are a popular and simple low-tech way to communicate.

that he was understood. The partner may also want to write down messages as they are composed so as not to forget. The board's size and the arrangement of items on the board are customized to the patient's range of movement.

Figure 8-1 illustrates two popular boards used by people with ALS. Your speech language pathologist can teach you how to use them, if needed. Both boards require that the patient be able to point to items on the board. Pointing may be done with a finger, a stylus attached to any part of the body, a laser pointer attached to a pair of glasses or head band, or with eye gaze. *Board A* is simple and portable. *Board B* is popular because it speeds up communication by providing whole words in addition to the alphabet. The core vocabulary chosen for this board represents the most commonly used words, which account for 50 percent of all words spoken. For ease of use, the words are color-coded and organized in alphabetical order within each word type (question words, time words, pronouns, verbs, etc.). A variety of effective communication boards also exist for patients who are unable to point.

Low-tech AAC systems are simple, inexpensive, portable, and reliable. Additionally, they provide excellent back-up to high-tech systems, so every high-tech user should have a low-tech system. The disadvantages of low-tech systems include the lack of speech output and partner dependency.

High-Tech Augmentative-Alternative Communication

High-tech AAC devices require electricity and actually produce speech. These devices can range from small, simple type-and-speak devices to fully functioning computers. Because people with ALS are generally literate and cognitively normal, they require devices that provide synthesized speech. Devices with synthesized speech are able to "speak" any message typed or entered into them. This allows users to generate their own messages on-the-spot and not just rely on messages prerecorded by others. Many patients with ALS use devices that produce both synthesized and recorded speech. They find that having some preprogrammed messages in their own voice (voice banking) or that of a friend makes the system feel more personalized. Recorded human speech is also frequently initially easier for unfamiliar communication partners to understand. For this reason, patients often use digitally recorded messages to introduce themselves, explain their communication device, and initiate phone conversations.

Another important feature of high-tech AAC systems is *rate enhancement*. Rate enhancement features speed up communication and cut down on the physical burden of forming messages. Choosing an AAC device with good rate enhancement features is essential, because communication

> Energy conservation is important for all patients with ALS.

with any AAC system is significantly slower than speech. Also, energy conservation is important for all patients with ALS. Some examples of the rate enhancement features available in high-tech AAC devices include:

- *Word prediction:* As the user begins to spell a word, the computer offers a list of common words that begin with that letter or series of letters. The user then simply selects the word in the list and the device types the entire word automatically.
- *Abbreviation expansion:* A short series of letters or numbers can be programmed to expand into an entire message. For example, each time a user types "NG," the AAC device will produce the message "I need my glasses, please."

- *Prestored phrases:* Messages, stories, comments, questions, and even speeches can be stored ahead of time and retrieved with the selection of a single key or button on an AAC device.

Even with all of these rate enhancement features, many people with ALS find that using their hands to operate the keyboard or touch screen becomes too difficult. Just as ALS may weaken the muscles for speech, it can also affect the muscles of the arms and hands. Assistive technology allows those with even severe hand and arm weakness to continue to use their computers and AAC systems.

What Is Assistive Technology?

Assistive technology is any strategy, equipment, modification, or technology that improves or restores ability to those with impaired function. The loss of arm and hand function has a major impact on communication. You

> Assistive technology is any strategy, equipment, modification, or technology that improves or restores ability to those with impaired function.

may find you can no longer write, dial and hold the phone, use the computer keyboard and mouse, write and receive e-mails, or type messages into your AAC device. Assistive technology allows you to once again perform these tasks, although often in very different ways.

Examples of assistive technology include use of:

- Large barrel pens that are easier to grasp.
- Using alternative areas of the body to operate standard or modified tools.
- Trackball or joystick in place of a mouse.
- Speech recognition software: A hands-free method in which your computer types as you dictate; special verbal commands allow you to use all computer applications and functions.

- Modified or single hand keyboards.
- Head-mouse: A wireless device that controls a computer cursor through head movement; a head-mouse used with a keyboard that is displayed on the screen allows hands-free typing.
- Eye gaze access: A device that allows typing and computer or AAC device access with the use of only eye movement.
- Switches: Sensors that can be activated by tiny movements of any part of the body; they can be used to control all of the operations of a computer or AAC device via scanning or Morse code.
- Scanning: A method used to select an item (e.g., letter, word, message, or icon) in which the items are presented or highlighted in a fixed sequence; the user waits until the desired item is presented and then chooses it by activating the switch.
- Morse code: A system for using Morse code with switches to spell messages and operate a computer; the Morse code is translated by computer software into letters or computer operations; Morse code must be learned but, once learned, it is much faster than switch scanning.

If you are experiencing hand weakness and having problems with writing or using your computer, talk to your occupational therapist or speech language pathologist about assistive technology. Also check the list of assistive technology Web sites at the end of this chapter.

A Perspective on Communication

For most of us, speech is an effortless process that we take for granted. The purpose of speech, of course, is communication. ALS may interfere with speech but there remain many options for communication. It is communication and not speech that is central to maintaining self determination, vital relationships, and a sense of identity and well-being. Various ideas for maintaining communication were presented in this chapter and many more exist. Using these methods requires patience, flexibility, and determination. You may need to alter your expectations as to how quickly you can communicate and simplify your communication style. Others may need to be educated as to how to communicate effectively with you and even be reminded at times that you want and expect to be included in conversations. Remember to share the particular communication challenges you are facing with your speech language pathologist. The rewards of finding solutions will be invaluable for you and your loved ones. Although speech may become impossible with ALS, communication should remain unlimited.

Resources

Speech Language Pathologist/AAC Specialist Referrals

American Speech and Hearing Association (ASHA)
(800) 368-8255
http://www.asha.org
(Site has a speech language pathologist Referral Database)

ALS Association (ALSA)
(818) 880-9007
http://www.alsa.org

Muscular Dystrophy Association (MDA)
(800) 572-1717
http://www.mdausa.org
(Site has information on MDA funding assistance for AAC and AT)

Augmentative-Alternative Communication Information

Communication Independence for the Neurologically Impaired (CINI)
http://www.cini.org
(Highlights: AAC Glossary, Guide to Commercially Available AAC/AT Devices, FAQ about ALS and Communication, Information on ordering Communication and Swallowing Solutions for the ALS/MND Community: A CINI Manual and Eye-Link Communication Boards)

Oregon and Southwest Washington ALS Chapter-AAC
http://www.alsa-or.org/adaptive/AAC
(Highlights: AAC Funding Options; ALS-AAC Stages; Information on Voice Recognition Software, Text-to-Speech Software, Onscreen Keyboard

Software, Dwell Click / Cursor Control Software, Head Controlled Mice, Eye Gaze Control, Brainwave Control)

Assistive Technology Information

ABLEDATA
http://www.abledata.com
(Highlights: Large Database of AT Equipment, Keyword Search for Equipment, Consumer Forum with AT Equipment Review, Articles on AT)

Microsoft Accessibility
http://www.microsoft.com/enable/at/default.aspx
(Highlights: Information on Accessibility Features Built into Windows, Guide to Types of AT Products, Catalog Search of AT Products, AT Tutorials)

Oregon and Southwest Washington ALS Chapter-Assistive Technology
http://www.alsa-or.org/adaptive/adaptive
(Highlights: Links to vendors by AT Type Including Voice Recognition Software, Switches, Mouse Emulation, AAC)

CHAPTER 9

Staying Mobile

This chapter discusses problems resulting from some degree of spasticity, balance, coordination difficulties, and weakness that can compromise the ability of people with ALS to function on a daily basis. Any one of these problems—or a combination—can make it hard for you to walk, get out of a chair, get dressed and ready for the day, write, or use your computer. This chapter will help you to maximize your abilities, minimize disability, prevent complications, and conserve energy.

Proactively Managing Mobility Issues

Physical changes, such as those associated with the progressive nature of ALS, can affect your ability to function independently and how you engage in social, personal, and professional activities. People often feel that they do not want to be seen in public if they cannot function independently. You may feel embarrassed and look at yourself differently if you need help to accomplish tasks that you previously took for granted. Equipment that may make tasks easier to accomplish is often rejected initially because of what it may represent. Often, the first response to needing equipment (such as a wheelchair) can be intimidating, giving rise to feelings of being "less than whole" and that you are giving in to the disease.

But there is another way to respond to these recommendations. In almost all stages of the disease, you can mitigate its effects on your life. Making good use of adaptive equipment or adapting the way you do things can allow you to be more independent. This can help you fight the disease and prevent you from giving in to it by helping you function in the world, rather than withdraw from those activities that bring you satisfaction and joy. The disease wins if you let your life be diminished by withdrawing from the world. This need not happen.

People often reject equipment designed to enhance mobility when it is first suggested, but accept it when they have had a chance to work out their feelings about the physical changes they are experiencing. One thing is certain: your functional ability will change over time, but so will your ability to adapt to those changes. You, your family, and your health care team need to have an ongoing dialogue about the use of equipment and adaptations. Recommendations from your team will range from simple to complex. You will need to weigh the costs and benefits of each solution. If the cost—either emotional or financial—outweighs the benefit, then it is not time for you to pursue that recommendation. You may come up with solutions to problems that your team has not thought of and they will want to hear about them. The reward for everyone involved is helping you achieve the greatest possible level of independence so that you can enjoy the things in life that are important to you.

Weakness and Spasticity

Muscle weakness in ALS results from a decreased number of functional motor nerve cells. This type of weakness differs from weakness that results from the disuse and deconditioning that might be experienced after an injury. Anyone who has ever had a broken arm will remember how much smaller their arm appeared when the cast was removed, and how their ability to perform activities with that arm was greatly reduced; however, with a program of exercise, the arm became stronger and resumed its previous strength.

When there is marked weakness as a result of lost or dysfunctional motor nerve cells, as is often the case in ALS, the nerves and muscles do not respond to increased exercise by getting substantially stronger. In fact, you may become more fatigued and even temporarily weaker in response to vigorous exercise. You may have noticed that you get very tired when you are using your weak arm or leg a lot. Most people find that if they stop an activity when they start to fatigue and rest briefly, they can then resume the activity.

Some degree of spasticity or muscle stiffness is common in people with upper motor neuron dysfunction. *Spasticity* is increased tension in a muscle that is especially obvious when that muscle is stretched. This stiffness can be painful and make even everyday tasks, such as walking and dressing, more difficult. Medication, exercise, physical therapy, and adaptive equipment (orthoses) can reduce spasticity, enhance coordination, improve function, and decrease pain. Spasticity may be increased by irritants, such as infection, extreme temperatures, constipation, pain, and anxiety, and you may want to avoid activities or irritants that increase your stiffness.

Exercise

Exercise is either a part of your everyday routine or an activity you are considering. Performing some form of exercise can be a simple and inexpensive addition to your daily routine that can yield major benefits throughout the disease process.

Mary is a 53-year-old woman with strong arms and legs who came to the clinic with speech and swallowing problems. She was participating in speech therapy sessions and had been doing voice exercises and a rigorous lip and tongue strengthening program. Mary found that after therapy, her speech was more slurred and she was too tired to eat meat at dinner. She had been walking 2 miles a day since she was diagnosed with hypertension 3 years before and wondered if this was contributing to her fatigue.

Comment: *Although Mary's speech therapy program was appropriate for someone who had suffered a stroke, it was not appropriate for someone with ALS. Performing excessive exercise involving the oral muscles caused her too much fatigue and increased her weakness in the evening. The speech pathologist at the clinic called her speech therapist in her home community and advised her to teach Mary compensation techniques for her slow, slurred speech and swallowing problems; the occupational therapist taught her oral stretching exercises that she could do* *at home. The physical therapist encouraged Mary to continue her walking program and indicated that they would reevaluate this program at her next appointment.*

People with ALS usually want to know what types and how much exercise is good for them. The answer is different for each person, depending on the nature and extent of their weakness and spasticity. The rule of thumb is that if performing an exercise does not fatigue or further weaken you, then you can and should do it.

Dan is a 56-year-old carpet and linoleum layer. His legs were strong, but he experienced some weakness and stiffness in his hands and shoulders. His hands would cramp when he used his tools in the early morning and late in the afternoon. He had no regular exercise program but was interested in starting up a routine.

Comments: *Dan talked with the occupational therapist at the clinic and developed a plan for modifying his work schedule to allow for periods of rest and activity for his arms at work. He was fitted for a hand splint that offered support to his thumbs and created less stress on his hands. Dan and his physical therapist discussed his interests, and he enrolled in a Tai Chi class at his local community college that helped him stretch his muscles and increased his flexibility.*

People with arm weakness should be alert for shoulder stiffness that could lead to "frozen shoulder" (*adhesive capsulitis*), which can be quite painful. Your physical and occupational therapists can help design a home program that incorporates specifics for your pattern of weakness. Conversely, people with weak legs and strong arms can do arm strengthening exercises but should gear their leg exercises toward stretching and maintaining strength. Your physical therapist can guide you in creating an appropriate routine.

Bob is a 46-year-old salesman who has strong but spastic legs. His walking had become stiffer and he sometimes felt as though he might fall, especially when walking in the backyard. He was a swimmer but found that the cold water at the pool seemed to increase his spasticity. He felt exhausted at the end of most days.

Comments: *A high degree of spasticity can diminish comfort and cause pain. Increased stiffness translates into increased energy needed to perform everyday activities. The physical therapist discussed switching to a warmer pool to decrease spasticity and encouraged Bob to do some aqua-therapy. The buoyancy of the water helped Bob move more freely, stretch adequately, and not have to fight gravity. She also gave him a stretching and range of motion program to do twice a day at home. Bob became more aware that walking on uneven surfaces can decrease stability. He and his therapist began exploring the use of an ankle foot orthosis to stabilize his ankle. Bob's ALS physician prescribed medication that helped to decrease his spasticity, especially at night.*

One way to decrease spasticity is by placing each of your freely moving joints into a position that stretches a spastic muscle—but does not cause pain—and holding that stretched position for at least a minute. This allows the muscle to slowly relax and decreases the stiffness. Your physical therapist can help you determine which muscles will most be helped by stretching and can train you and your caregiver in the positioning that will give you the best stretch. Ask your physical therapist to instruct you in range of motion exercises that move joints but do not hold a stretch for any specified length of time.

It may also help to use orthotics to counteract spasticity and maintain a more natural position of a joint. All of these interventions will help prevent joints from freezing up into an unnatural position.

Getting Up from a Seated Position

Mild muscle weakness may make it difficult to get up from a chair. Generally, raising the hips higher than the knees can make it easier to stand up. An inexpensive example of simple equipment is to place a 2- to 3-inch thick cushion in a chair. This can make getting up easier and the cushion can be moved from chair to chair. You might consider raising the height of a favorite chair with blocks or commercially available chair leg lifters. Many people find it helpful to purchase an electric lift recliner chair that will allow you to rise to a standing position with the use of an electric control. These chairs do most of the work necessary to get you into a standing position, or if help is still needed, they can greatly reduce the amount of effort that your caregiver needs to expend. Although more costly, this type of chair looks like any other recliner you would find in the living room and has the added benefit that the electric control can also be used to recline the chair.

Using the same principle, you may find that elevating the toilet seat helps you to be independent in the bathroom. A variety of seats can be attached directly to the toilet; your physical therapist or occupational therapist can help you decide which one will work well with the toilet in your home. Some people prefer to have a commode chair (a portable seat on wheels with a cutout for toileting needs) that can be pushed away from the toilet easily or used in the bedroom to decrease long walks to the bathroom at night or in other rooms, as needed.

If getting up and standing unassisted is challenging but you have good arm strength and balance, you may be able to use a sliding board to transfer independently or with minimal assistance. These boards are made of plastic or wood and have a smooth surface that, when placed under your buttocks, allows you to use your arms to push across the surface and onto another chair. Mechanical lifters are available if more assistance is required; they can be used to move you from bed to chair or commode with the help of a caregiver.

Walking

When walking requires a lot of energy or becomes unsafe, you will need to consider a more practical means to accomplish this goal. People with ALS often develop a condition called *foot drop* in which the toes of the affected foot touch the ground before the heel. The effort to lift the foot high enough to clear the ground is enormous and exhausting, and the ensuing poor balance increases the likelihood of a fall. A simple solution is a plastic or carbon graphite ankle foot orthosis that fits into a shoe and can pick up the foot and allow it to follow through in the normal heel-to-toe pattern. The physical therapist and orthotist will design a type of ankle foot orthosis that will not aggravate any spasticity present and will help decrease fatigue and increase stability (Figure 9-1).

Your therapist may recommend an additional device to increase stability when an ankle foot orthosis alone cannot compensate for weakness. She may advise a cane or forearm Lofstrand crutch if your arm strength is good. Having an additional point of contact with the ground will help to maintain your balance.

If you have noticed that you walk more easily and quickly when using a shopping cart at the supermarket, a four-wheeled walker may help

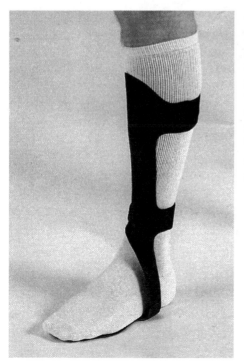

FIGURE 9-1

An ankle foot orthosis is a lightweight ankle brace made of polypropylene or carbon graphite. It is designed to compensate for a foot drop by preventing the foot from turning or the toe from catching. The orthotic inserts into the shoe under the sole and comes up to mid-calf to stabilize the ankle.

Camp-Toe OFF™ – Rehabilitation Orthosis

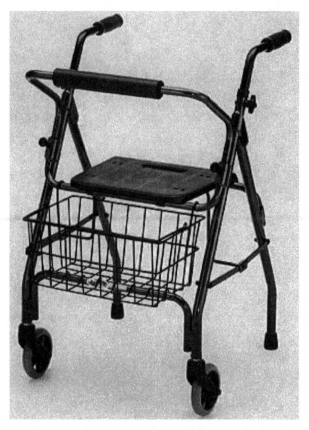

FIGURE 9-2

Four-wheeled walker with brakes and a seat improves stability and safety of walking.

Cruiser II Walker – NOVA – Ortho-med, Inc.

a great deal. These lightweight devices are easily folded and placed in a car, and have the advantage of having brakes for control and a seat (Figure 9-2). Most people with ALS find that if they sit down for a few minutes when they begin to tire while walking, they can get back up and continue walking quite easily. If you continue walking past the point of fatigue, getting back up and continuing walking becomes more daunting. You may find that you can walk further and faster if you have wheels to smooth out your walking, handles to lean on to support your trunk muscles and prop up your posture, and a seat with you. There are many different types of four-wheeled walkers, and your therapist can help you decide which type will best compensate for your particular weakness and pattern of walking. An additional bonus is that the seat or basket can be used to carry things from one room to another or home from the market.

Although imagining yourself in a wheelchair is difficult, many people with ALS find that the intermittent use of a lightweight portable wheelchair for long distances is a boon to their social life. They come in particularly handy in places such as airports, museums, or malls, where there are long distances to walk and very crowded conditions that can easily knock you off balance. Being chauffeured to a restaurant leaves you with enough energy to enjoy your meal and the company. You can transfer out of the wheelchair and sit in a regular chair once you arrive.

Once you have conquered any anxiety that you have about using a wheelchair and realize how much more energy you have for doing things that are enjoyable, you may want to consider a power chair. Your independence can increase dramatically once you begin to use a power chair. Not only can you power yourself to anywhere you want to go, but you can also change your position for comfort—all without asking anyone else to help you. Do make sure that you get the advice of your physical therapist and occupational therapist before buying one, because there is nothing more frustrating than spending your scarce insurance dollars on an expensive power wheelchair that works for you now but that cannot be modified when you have a slight change in your abilities.

Arm and Shoulder Weakness

People with ALS are prone to elbow, forearm, wrist, and hand weakness, which can make it hard to manipulate utensils for work, self care, and leisure activities. Many useful devices can make these tasks more manageable. Your occupational therapist can show you inexpensive simple solutions such as wrist splints; button and zipper hooks; foam for building up eating utensils, pens, and toothbrushes; lightweight shavers and toothbrushes; adapted dental floss holders; shoelaces that you do not have to tie; playing card holders; and many other gadgets that will help simplify your life. You might find that mobile arm supports that allow easy horizontal and vertical movements make both computer work and eating easier.

You will find that balancing work with rest periods (either a nap or resting a joint or muscle group) allows you to get far more done than using up all of your energy at once early in the day. Organizing your work areas

A

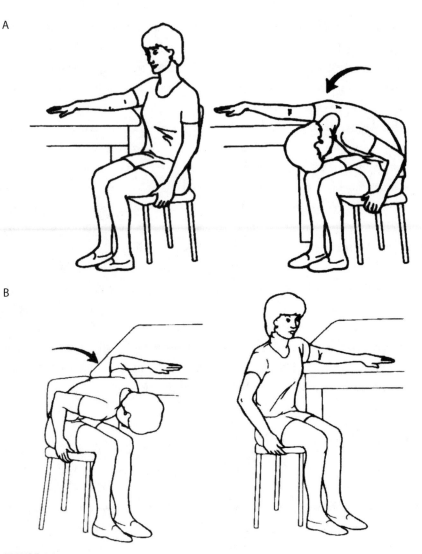

B

FIGURE 9-3

Mobility
Shoulder Flexion (A):
    Arm on table
    Lean forward and scoot chair back so you feel a stretch
    Hold 1 to 2 minutes
Shoulder Outward Rotation (B):
    Arm on table as you sit sideways next to table
    Elbow bent about 70 degrees
    Lean forward so that you feel a stretch in your shoulder
    Hold at *mild* stretch for 1 to 2 minutes

by placing articles between your wrist and shoulder cuts down on the effort needed, as does sitting to accomplish work instead of standing.

Shoulder weakness usually leads to a frozen shoulder unless stretching exercises are performed regularly to prevent this painful condition (Figure 9-3).

Taking Control

Walking is one of the basic sources of autonomy. Mobility gives you the opportunity to move towards pleasurable activities and withdraw from less comfortable situations. Anything—a sprained ankle, bunions, or fatigue—that decreases mobility affects your sense of power and control over the world. Knowing beforehand about ways to deal with the often inevitable problems with mobility that ALS brings can help you deal with them proactively. Committing to fully living with this disease and taking control in whatever manner feasible is an act of courage and hope. Each decision you make over the course of this disease makes the next decision easier to make. Encourage your loved ones and your health care team to offer their advice and help in your decision-making process.

CHAPTER 10

Breathing and Sleeping

In this chapter, we will discuss how ALS can affect the muscles involved in breathing. There is only one good reason for this discussion: there is so very much we can do to help manage the breathing difficulties associ-

> There is so much we can do to help manage breathing difficulties in ALS.

ated with ALS. Some aspects of these problems may initially seem overwhelming or even frightening, but we urge you to continue reading and remind yourself that there is treatment available to improve your breathing and sleeping. Breathing difficulties may have been of concern, but hopefully by the end of this chapter you will appreciate that there are always solutions to respiratory problems.

Many muscle groups are involved in normal breathing. They are called the *respiratory muscles* and they include the muscles of the tongue, throat, palate, neck, rib cage, abdomen, and diaphragm (Figure 10-1).

Sometimes ALS-related muscle weakness results in difficulties with clearing secretions from the airways. Patients have more difficulty with bronchial infections when this occurs because they are unable to adequately cough and sneeze to clear phlegm. Various devices can provide assistance during this period:

- A nebulizer can deliver inhaled medicines to open the airways and break up phlegm.
- A special (ABI) vest vibrates to raise secretions from the base of the lungs up to the mouth where they can be eliminated.
- A *cofflator* (also known as an *insufflator-exsufflator*) is a special suction device that can be used over the nose or mouth to assist with

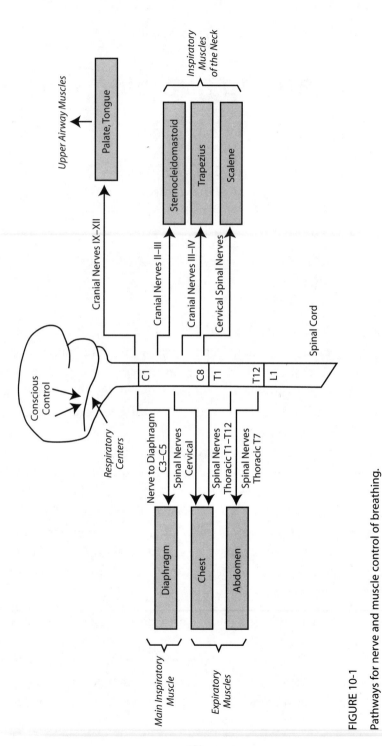

FIGURE 10-1

Pathways for nerve and muscle control of breathing.

sneezing or coughing and help evacuate phlegm from the nasal or bronchial air passages.

These devices help people with ALS recover from colds, flu, or pneumonia more quickly; they also help prevent hospitalization.

Although respiratory muscle weakness is common in ALS and occurs in everyone eventually during the course of the disease, many patients are totally unaware of the weakening of their respiratory system. It is important for doctors caring for people with ALS to watch very closely for the earliest indication of respiratory muscle weakness, because weakness of breathing muscles may develop over a relatively long period of time without any obvious symptoms. This involves a thorough discussion of symptoms with your doctor as well as performing various tests of muscle and lung function while in the office for an ALS visit. The most commonly performed test of lung function in ALS clinics is called the *forced vital capacity*, which measures the total lung volume that you are able to forcibly exhale (breathe out). This test is very sensitive to changes in muscle strength, although it is not a direct measure of respiratory muscle strength. In very rare cases, shortness of breath may be an early sign of ALS, although typically, people with ALS do not develop breathing problems until the disease is quite advanced.

Symptoms of Weakness of Breathing Muscles

In the early stages of ALS, most people are free of any breathing difficulties or may have shortness of breath only on exertion. Those with weakness that involves the muscles of the diaphragm may become short of breath after eating a large meal or when lying flat on their backs because the contents of the stomach may move up into the lung space. Many lung function tests performed at the clinic may be normal when respiratory muscle strength is only mildly weakened.

As respiratory muscle weakness becomes more advanced, people with ALS may still not feel short of breath, especially if they also have weakness of arm and leg muscles that prevents them from moving excessively. People with ALS may spend most of their day in a more sedentary lifestyle, and they may never be aware of any air hunger during waking hours. The first sign of difficulty may occur during sleep, although even then, people are typically not aware of any shortness of breath, but simply note that they wake up more frequently during the night for a variety of reasons—because the cat is making noises, they need to go to the bathroom, it requires more effort to roll over, etc. In reality, they may be waking up because their level of sleep is lighter because their depth of breathing is shallower. The next morning, they may not feel well rested and may feel as though their energy level is dragging during the day. In addition, some people may notice that their voice is softer, their cough is less effective in clearing their throat, or they breathe more rapidly. All these changes are quite subtle. The most important study that can evaluate whether ALS is weakening the muscles of respiration and disturbing sleep is a special study known as a *polysomnogram.*

A polysomnogram is performed while you sleep. It records many different processes, such as air movement through the nose, chest movement, stomach movement, the level of oxygen in the blood, and brain and muscle electrical activity. This test can identify the specific causes of disturbed sleep. People with ALS who awaken multiple times because of weak breathing may not be consciously aware of it, but this test can detect the problem, and the underlying cause of the sleep disturbance can then be corrected.

A 56-year-old woman with a 2-year history of ALS complained of difficulty staying asleep at night and the need to nap during the day because of fatigue. She fell asleep at night with no difficulty, but would awaken every hour after about 2 a.m. She denied any shortness of breath but felt that she woke up because of discomfort in her legs and back due to muscle weakness and her inability to roll over in bed. She refused to believe that her sleep problems could be due to respiratory involvement because her breathing was quite comfortable; however, she did agree to a sleep study. The polysomnogram documented that she had low oxygen levels prior to each time she woke up and that her low oxygen resulted in light sleep, which then led to her arous-

al and her awareness of discomfort in her legs and back. During the second stage of the sleep study, she was fitted with a nasal mask attached to a breathing machine (a noninvasive pressure ventilator), which guaranteed that she continued to take deep breaths even while asleep. Her oxygen levels no longer dropped when she used this noninvasive ventilator and she was able to stay asleep the rest of the night.

Comment: *This case illustrates how the earliest sign of respiratory weakness may be disturbed sleep and the resulting daytime sleepiness and fatigue, even though daytime breathing function is quite good.*

Managing Respiratory Infections

Acute breathing difficulties from infection may become severe, especially if you have other diseases in addition to ALS that can affect breathing, such as asthma, emphysema, heart disease, marked obesity, blood clots, or pneumonia. Even a viral infection can cause severe problems with cough and secretions that can become exhausting for people with respiratory muscle weakness due to ALS. We recommend a vaccine to protect you against common strains of bacterial pneumonia (pneumococcal) and yearly flu vaccines. When respiratory infections cannot be avoided, they should be treated aggressively and early with inhalation treatments—and in some cases with antibiotics—to help clear secretions out of the airway passages. Respiratory infection should never be ignored in the hope that it will clear up by itself. Most infections can be treated very successfully if caught early, before you are exhausted.

Sleep and Respiratory Muscle Compromise

Sleep is the ideal time to detect the earliest changes in breathing function, especially during the stage of dream sleep, which is a very active stage in terms of heart and other body function demands. Depression of oxygen levels in the blood during sleep can lead to serious health consequences if it remains uncorrected. These include chronic lung problems, heart failure, and eventually death. Warning signs that sleep problems are reaching crit-

> Sleep is the ideal time to detect the earliest changes in breathing function.

ically dangerous and life-threatening proportions include morning headaches, excessive daytime sleepiness, mental confusion, overwhelming fatigue even after resting, and leg swelling. It is important to remember that the degree of breathing muscle weakness with ALS may not be proportional to the degree of weakness of other muscles—arms and legs may be relatively strong, while breathing is weak; all of the muscles that control limb and breathing may be weak; or there may be any combination thereof. Regular visits to an ALS clinic (approximately every 3 months) to discuss how you are feeling, along with a few simple tests and an occasional sleep study, can identify whether you are at risk for breathing difficulties and treat problems before any crisis occurs.

Instituting Noninvasive Mechanical Breathing Assistance

As noted above, once sleep-related symptoms due to low levels of oxygen in the blood are identified, a polysomnogram may be useful in identifying those who fail to breathe deeply enough during sleep. A simpler study called an *oxygen saturation test*, which can be done in your own home, measures your oxygen level during sleep via a probe taped to your finger. Most healthy people spend 90 percent of the night with oxygen levels above 89 percent and do not drop below 90 percent. Therefore, this simple overnight oxygen saturation study provides a lot of information and indicates whether a longer and more expensive sleep study (the polysomnogram) might be necessary. These tests help to clarify whether you would benefit from breathing assistance during sleep.

Once it has been confirmed that you do indeed have shallow breathing at night and that oxygen levels are low, there are treatments available to correct the problem. The most popular treatment is the *noninvasive ventilator*. This device delivers pressurized room air into the lungs, guaranteeing a deep breath with each breath you take. The air can be delivered through a variety of masks or tubes (whichever you prefer). Some fit into the nostrils; some fit over the nostrils; some fit like a mask over the nose alone; others fit over the mouth alone; and still others fit over the nose and mouth. They are designed for all face and nose shapes so that they are comfortable and can be kept on for hours while sleeping.

The idea is to use noninvasive ventilation while resting or sleeping, to rest the breathing muscles and support the body with a good oxygen supply for 4 to 8 hours. The mask and ventilator are removed after waking up. This is not considered life support because you are not attached to the machine; you simply put it on at night as you would a hat and take it off again in the morning. By contrast, a ventilator with a *tracheostomy*, a tube placed surgically in the throat, is an invasive option that is regarded as a life support measure. This option is not commonly chosen by people with ALS because of the increased burden and cost of care.

Noninvasive ventilation restores low blood oxygen levels, reestablishes normal sleep patterns, and greatly prolongs the lives of people with ALS. In addition, people report improved energy and a sense of well-being. Noninvasive ventilation has done more to enhance the quality of life and the life expectancy of patients with ALS than any other drug or treatment.

CHAPTER 11

Thinking and Behavioral Changes

Susan Woolley Levine, PhD

For many years, ALS was considered to be a disease that affected only the motor system. The mind was considered to be spared from any changes, remaining totally intact. However, we have learned more recently that this is not the case for some people with ALS. Researchers have discovered that changes in cognition (thinking) can sometimes even occur early in the course of the disease. These changes are generally very mild and do not cause patients much concern. Common difficulties include problems in finding the right word or making decisions as effectively as they did previously.

Patients and their families have not been consistently informed about this potential issue because it was not recognized until recently. Patients and family members can better identify common cognitive and behavioral changes when they are educated about them. Early identification can lead to effective treatment and accommodations, which will minimize the impact of any changes on their daily life.

This chapter discusses the common cognitive and behavioral changes seen in ALS, how they differ from normal, age-related cognitive changes and the changes associated with other diseases (such as Alzheimer's disease), and what can be done about them.

What Is Cognition?

The word *cognition* refers to thinking, knowing, perceiving, and understanding information. Our cognitive systems are highly complex and involve many areas of the brain, yet we process information constantly without exerting much conscious effort at all. Different aspects of cognition include attention, concentration, memory, language, organization of thoughts, planning, and decision-making. We need to pay attention and concentrate on what is happening around us in order to understand and learn. Attention and concentration are the gateway functions to more complex abilities, including *memory*, which is a complex process that involves imprinting information into the brain, filing it away, and retrieving it when needed again.

Some of our normal thought processes involve concentrating on and learning information, which then allows us to plan, analyze, and make decisions. These and other tasks are sometimes referred to as *executive functions*. Like a business executive who is in charge of many different responsibilities, our brains have an executive function that coordinates the processing, integration, and analysis of a lot of information. The part of our brain that controls these functions is called the *frontal lobes*; it is also involved with judgment, insight, and self-awareness. This is the same part of the brain in which voluntary control over the motor system resides.

We all have strengths and weaknesses when it comes to thought processes. Some people can organize a grocery list in their head without notes, while others struggle to remember the name of a new doctor. The brain is complex and resilient, and its effectiveness can be affected by many factors.

Normal Age-Related Cognitive Changes

By now you are probably thinking of the times when your cognition was less than ideal, whether it involved feeling absent-minded during a conversation or forgetting why you entered a room. As frustrating and worrisome as these moments can be, they are generally quite normal as we become older. For example, we become more vulnerable to distraction (background noises or other interruptions), making it harder to pay attention and hold information in our minds, such as new phone numbers. It also becomes harder to think of certain words. The problem of coming up with the word we want becomes much more common as we get older, but most people will eventually recall the word they are searching for if they relax.

The speed of the thinking process begins to slow down as we age. There is a "use-it-or-lose-it" quality to our thinking in that irrelevant facts or events are more easily forgotten than information we need and use on a regular basis. *Prospective* memory (remembering to remember) becomes harder, but we actually enhance this type of memory when we use notes or other reminders. Despite assumptions to the contrary, making notes or leaving reminders for yourself can help your memory and mental organization. You can also strengthen your thinking when you pursue intellectual stimulation and active learning, such as reading or enrolling in an educational class.

Cognitive Changes in People with ALS

Some of you are now probably breathing a sigh of relief, knowing that the occasional cognitive glitches that you experience are not a clear sign of impending doom. However, you and your family still need to be aware of possible disease-related changes in thought processes.

Research studies have revealed that one-third to one-half of patients with ALS experiences some changes in thinking. The evaluation of these symptoms is complicated by the muscle weakness and/or speech impair-

> One-third to one-half of patients with ALS experiences some changes in thinking.

ment of ALS. However, using brain imaging and cognitive tests, doctors have discovered regions in the brains of some patients that reflect impairment. These changes are often very subtle and may not be noticed without medical tests.

Although many questions still remain, it appears that patients with speech or swallowing difficulty may have cognitive difficulties earlier on in the disease when compared with the patients whose weakness begins in the limbs. Patients with speech and swallowing problems are more likely to develop cognitive dysfunction over time when compared with others.

However, patients whose ALS begins in the limbs may also develop cognitive difficulties.

A number of different types of changes in thinking can be associated with ALS. For example, concentrating can be more difficult for some people. *Concentration* refers to the ability to maintain a sustained focus on a task, such as mental calculations. It not only involves paying attention, but also holding the necessary information in mind in order to manipulate or modify it. You may have difficulty shifting your attention from one thing to another or considering two ideas/perspectives at the same time. In other instances, some patients may have trouble with planning, organizing information, making decisions, showing good judgment, or having insight about how they are doing. Similarly, the ability to self-monitor or benefit from feedback from others may not be as good as it once was. Finally, your *language output*, including the ability to think of certain words, may change.

These cognitive changes are often very subtle and may not be identified without specialized psychological testing to assess various cognitive functions. Usually, people with ALS do not complain of any cognitive problems. However, sometimes an observant, concerned family member notices problems with paying attention, following conversations, or organizing thoughts. Others may notice reduced talkativeness or a change in the amount or type of words used, independent of actual speech problems.

A 60-year-old woman with ALS denied having problems with cognition, yet her spouse described deterioration in her ability to communicate. She was losing at Scrabble™, a game she always used to win. She also started getting lost while driving and had trouble managing her finances. Neurocognitive testing revealed changes in language, reflecting how difficult it was for her to think of words. The testing also discovered changes that reflected problems with her ability to organize her thoughts and follow through on them.

Comment: *Family members can sometimes identify cognitive changes in patients with ALS that the patient may not be aware of or may not be willing to disclose.*

Behavioral Changes Associated with ALS

The changes that can cause cognitive problems in the brains of people with ALS can also cause changes in personality and behavior. Unlike the cognitive changes, which are often subtle, these behavioral changes tend to be

> It is often a family member who first notices personality changes.

more prominent. As with cognitive changes, it is often a family member who first notices personality changes. That is why it is important to have friends or family members involved in your care. They can lend important perspectives as to your abilities and behavioral styles before the ALS diagnosis that may differ from what you report or present to medical staff.

Several types of behavioral changes can be seen in ALS. One pattern is characterized by *apathy*, a lack of initiative or interest in life. Individuals suffering from apathy have difficulty being spontaneous and appear to have low motivation. Apathy is often confused with depression and can be hard to identify because the physical changes and fatigue of ALS make it harder for patients to initiate conversations or movements. Given the motor slowness and diminished speech output, people with ALS may be labeled and treated as depressed without further exploration into other problems. Usually the difference is that people who are depressed feel sad and tearful, whereas apathetic patients do not necessarily experience significant changes in mood.

Another type of behavioral change—one seen less frequently in people with ALS—involves the loss of a person's usual and appropriate sense of social inhibition or a lowering of self-control. Occasionally patients with ALS may lack social graces even though they were previously very socially aware and well controlled. Individuals who lose their sense of social appropriateness may become hyperactive, extremely irritable, or emotionally labile.

A 40-year-old man with ALS was described by his wife and caregiver as easily agitated, distractable, and very irritable. Neuropsychological testing revealed a clear change in personality and problems with concentration and generating new ideas. This information helped the treatment team and his family develop ways of interacting with him that minimized his irritability and distraction. He was also given medication that helped both his thinking and behavior.

Of course, everyone may have days when they are more irritable or less polite than usual. This type of behavior is only considered a problem when it occurs on a more consistent basis and disrupts daily life.

More Advanced Deficits—Frontotemporal Dementia

The impairment is more extensive in some people with ALS and fits with a profile known as *frontotemporal dementia* (FTD). FTD produces a combination of more severe cognitive and behavioral/personality changes than those discussed above. The beginning stages of FTD can seem the same as the milder, ALS-related changes. Over time, however, the cognitive problems become worse. For example, patients with FTD may have significant problems with language skills, leaving them unable to communicate effectively with others. The behavioral problems associated with FTD can become quite serious. Patients with FTD may have little control over their impulses, becoming aggressive or explosive. Conversely, they may become severely withdrawn and apathetic. FTD causes patients to have significant difficulty functioning in normal social situations or living independently. This condition is progressively disabling, but treatments including medications to enhance thinking and improve behavior can be provided if it is identified early. Accommodations, such as techniques to manage difficult behaviors, can also be made so that the effects of the disease are minimized.

ALS Is Different from Alzheimer's Disease

People often think of Alzheimer's disease (AD) when they hear the word *dementia*. The changes that occur in ALS and FTD are *not* the same as

AD. Alzheimer's disease primarily disturbs memory, but it also affects many other cognitive functions. Individuals with AD have great difficulty learning and retaining new information, and eventually they forget their loved ones, where they live, and even their own name. Unlike AD,

> There is no evidence that ALS increases the risk of Alzheimer's disease.

the changes associated with ALS generally do not affect memory. People with ALS may have slight problems with memory because their concentration may be worse, making it more difficult for a lot of information to be absorbed. However, once the information gets in, patients with ALS generally do not forget it. Of course, some elderly patients with ALS may also have AD, but no clear relationship exists between the two diseases. In other words, there is no evidence that ALS increases the risk of AD.

Other Factors Affecting Cognition

As mentioned before, many things can affect cognition and behavior. Some of the most important are depression, anxiety, stress, alcohol, and medications. These are problems that anyone can suffer from, and luckily there are many ways to successfully deal with them.

Depression refers to feeling sad, down, or tearful. These feelings can be quite normal if they occur intermittently, but if they last for 2 weeks or more and do not seem to lessen, then something more significant might be happening. It may be helpful to talk to your doctor if you notice this in yourself or a family member.

Depression not only affects your mood and your ability to complete your usual, daily responsibilities, but it can also impair your cognition. For example, it can become much harder to concentrate, make decisions, or initiate activities. These problems may sound similar to the problems associated with ALS. This is why it is important to talk to your physician if you suspect that something is wrong. That way, he can more accurately identify what is happening and treat it.

The wife of a 56-year-old man with ALS reported to her husband's doctor that he seemed distracted and did not pay attention in conversations. He denied having these problems. Although the doctor wondered about the possibility of cognitive difficulties, the evaluation by the psychologist revealed that the patient was depressed. He was started on medications and when he returned 2 months later, his attention and concentration had improved, as had his mood and interaction with others.

Similarly, anxiety may affect mood and alter thinking. Anxious people tend to be very distracted by their worries, which get in the way of attention and concentration. Stress, which is sometimes considered to be related to anxiety, refers to physical, mental, or emotional tension. This can also make it very difficult for us to pay attention or learn new information.

Depression, anxiety, and stress can all cause sleep problems and fatigue, which make it more challenging to be at our best. Sleep allows our brains to organize all of the new information we took in during the day. Thus, without enough sleep, we cannot pay attention or learn as well. This is one reason why mechanical breathing assistance (see Chapter 10) helps people with ALS who have nighttime breathing difficulties feel better. Not only does breathing improve, but patients feel more clearheaded because they sleep more.

Another factor that can affect cognition and behavior is excessive alcohol use. Although many people enjoy a glass of wine or a beer now and then, others tend to drink too much alcohol and may use it to cope with problems or escape their worries. Although this may seem helpful in the short-term, its effectiveness is fleeting and can lead to many problems. Excessive alcohol can disrupt normal sleep patterns and has other damaging effects on our bodies over time, including our brains. It is recommended that a doctor be consulted if questions arise as to how much may be too much.

Finally, certain medications can cause subtle changes in the efficiency of our thinking. The side effects of some medications may make it harder to concentrate or make quick decisions. Tell your doctor if you suspect that the onset of cognitive changes coincided with the start of a new medication.

Identifying Cognitive and Behavioral Changes

Neuropsychological or neurocognitive testing typically involves paper and pencil tests or verbal tests. It may also involve a psychological assessment to measure some of the factors previously discussed (i.e., depression, anxiety, stress, sleep, and substance use). The results are compared with scores of other people of the same age, gender, and education level. This comparison helps distinguish between age-related changes and those associated with ALS. There are patterns in the test scores that are unique to ALS and FTD that help doctors identify problems.

Treating Cognitive and Behavioral Problems

The primary mode of treatment for cognitive and behavioral changes is with medication. Several types of medications can be used for this purpose. Some help people feel more alert, which helps with depression and apathy. Other medications are targeted specifically for problems with thinking,

> The primary mode of treatment for cognitive and behavioral changes is with medication.

although they have not been widely studied yet in the ALS population. There are also medications that can help if you are feeling anxious, socially inappropriate, or irritable. Your doctor has many options to choose from and, if one medication does not work, others can be considered.

Another way to manage these changes is to modify the environment. For people with cognitive changes, it is helpful to make their home structured and organized so that there is minimal confusion or distraction. You can establish specific locations for frequently used things such as keys, wallet, or glasses. Occupational therapists can be very helpful in providing resources and strategies for adapting your home. Another means of adding structure includes organizing daily information by using a calendar or notes.

Communication with individuals who are cognitively compromised or behaviorally impaired is another important issue. It is important to minimize distractions—for example, in-depth conversations in the middle of a shopping mall are not recommended. Distractions can cause some individuals to lose their ability to focus on a topic, causing agitation or irritability. Also, try to avoid giving too much information when talking to people with cognitive problems, as this may lead to information overload and decreased concentration. It is generally more helpful to ask yes/no questions (Are you happy?) rather than open-ended ones (How do you feel?). It is also important to maintain a positive tone when communicating. These are just a few examples; many more ideas can be provided by your health care team, and these can be tailored to meet your specific situation and needs.

Summary

Cognitive and behavioral changes are now recognized as fairly common occurrences in ALS. These changes often go unnoticed because they can be mild and make minimal impact on day-to-day life. Although some changes can make interpersonal interactions more challenging, there are several ways to treat them so the impact is minimized. A number of conditions can cause thinking and behavioral problems and many of these are completely treatable. We strongly encourage you and your family members to openly discuss cognitive, personality, or behavioral changes with your health care team so that interventions and accommodations can be made.

CHAPTER 12

Pallative Care

The term *palliative care* refers to the practice of medicine to control and manage symptoms to improve the quality of life for a person who is suffering from a disease that cannot be cured. It is not always the same as hospice care—which is palliative care offered at the final stages of life—

> Palliative care treats the person who suffers with ALS, not the ALS itself.

although it is an essential part of good hospice care. Palliative care treats the person who suffers with ALS, not the ALS itself. People are viewed within the context of their family, community, ethnicity, friendships, and spirituality. The focus is on allowing people to spend the remaining portion of their lives the way they choose to spend it, unhindered by pain, depression, unnecessary medical concerns, or despair.

Robert, a 42-year-old man suffering with advanced ALS, realized that his ALS was progressing very rapidly in spite of Rilutek®. Participation in the ALS research trial was becoming more exhausting for him. He asked his research doctor to tell him frankly how much time he had left because he and his wife, Jane, had experiences that were very important for them to share while he still had sufficient energy to participate. At first, Robert's doctor tried to encourage them by saying that new drugs might be available any day to cure his disease, but after what seemed like hours, they finally had a painful and truthful discussion. The doctor agreed that the progression of Robert's disease was indeed very rapid—unusually so—and that it might be advisable to consult with a palliative care physician. The next week, Robert and Jane returned to the ALS center to meet with the palliative care doctor. Her emphasis was different. She was more interested in them as a couple, their children, their backgrounds, and their plans for the future. She was also interested in day-to-day symptoms, such as quality of sleep, appetite, energy level, and practical solutions to problems. She encouraged Robert to finish the research trial but to change his priorities so that his life plans with Jane would become central.

When Jane asked how long Robert had to live, the palliative care doctor answered: "Most people with ALS live about 2 to 3 years after they are diagnosed, although I have seen exceptions. Some have diseases that progress slower, others faster. Unfortunately, yours seems to be a fast-moving disease. Although I cannot tell you exactly how long you have to live, I would say it is on the shorter end of the spectrum. However, I can promise you that I will not abandon you. There is much I can do for you, even if we are powerless to cure your ALS. I am confident that we can respect your wishes as to how you want to live the rest of your life and we can make sure you do not have worrisome symptoms. Are there more questions you have for me about your disease?"

Robert and Jane asked many more questions and felt they received honest answers. They cried, but they felt relieved. They left the clinic that day feeling much clearer about his disease and their future. They began to make plans again.

Physicians sometimes unintentionally abandon people with ALS by failing to tell patients the truth about the severity of their disease. However, by telling the truth about the severity of the ALS, physicians can help patients to: (1) manage their expectations for the future realistically; (2) be more compliant with treatment plans; and (3) paradoxically, cultivate hope in a new vision of the future. Although few ALS centers have a designated palliative care physician, all have physicians who are trained in palliative care practices. A person with ALS who wishes to be treated more holistically need only make those desires known. Consult the Web sites cited at the end of this chapter for help finding a physician with experience in palliative care.

Later, when Jane asked Robert how he felt about having a second doctor involved in his care, he said, "I kind of like having my research doctor focus on 'the cure' and my palliative care doctor focus on me."

Many months passed and Robert and Jane worked through many issues with their children, elderly parents, and brothers and sisters. They felt that they became closer to their entire extended family—old grievances were aired and they received a lot of loving support from friends. Although never very religious in the past, this experience led them to seek answers to questions about the meaning of suffering and the impermanence of life, and the significance of life itself. Together they began a spiritual journey. By listening to books on tape and reading material from different religions, they learned to accept life with its disappointments and feared death less.

Robert's disease progressed very rapidly, as they had expected, and soon he required total care. Luckily, Jane had many loving people around to help, but still the main burden fell on her and she was exhausted. At the next ALS clinic appointment, the palliative care doctor spent more time checking Jane—whose blood pressure was high—than Robert who was comfortable and well cared for. Jane was urged to see her family doctor and then to take a weekend off with her children while Robert's parents cared for him. Jane returned home refreshed and ready to continue seeing Robert through his disease.

Eventually, Robert's breathing became shallower and it was necessary to move him once or twice an hour to keep him comfortable. Hospice care was discussed with the palliative care physician and the decision was made to start hospice to provide more in-home support. The hospice intake nurse came to the home and explained the services that would be provided. She explained that Robert's survival was now expected to be less than 6 months and that relieving his physical, mental, emotional, and spiritual discomfort was the main concern.

Robert and Jane were prepared for this and agreed that care and comfort were what they wanted—neither of them wanted Robert to go through more medical procedures. They both wanted Robert to die comfortably at home surrounded by his family. They signed the hospice papers and agreed to call hospice in case of an emergency. They were relieved to hear that their ALS palliative care doctor would still be managing Robert's care. After the administrative matters were taken care of, the hospice nurse performed a medical history, again asking many questions about the family and conducting a short physical exam that included checking Robert's temperature, respirations, heart rate, and blood pressure. She took note of all the medications Robert required and informed him that hospice would be providing him with his medications from now on. In addition, she would check on him once or twice a week and a home health aide would come 3 days a week to help bathe and feed him. A social worker made visits to Robert and Jane as well as each of the children. He talked openly but warmly about being prepared for Robert's death. He also listened to how the children were adjusting and let Jane know that one of the children was having a little extra difficulty. At Robert's request, a chaplain came by who was very knowledgeable about world religions, and he and Robert and Jane had a fascinating discussion one afternoon regarding the views of death and the afterlife of many major religions from reincarnation to resurrection. He recommended many interesting books to further Robert and Jane's spiritual quest.

With all of the different people from hospice visiting daily, Jane felt less alone and less afraid of losing Robert. She had noticed that Robert was becoming much less interested in the family and was spending more and more time quietly resting in bed. He ate very little and had less energy, even for conversation with her. She found it hard to let him go and sometimes she felt angry that he had not fought harder to hold on to life. The hospice people explained that Robert was going through a very natural process of separating from this world in order to attach himself to the next—however he envisioned that next world to be. They further explained that the greatest gift Jane could give Robert at this time in his illness was the gift of a loving release from this world and his life of suffering with ALS. It took several more weeks but, ultimately, as Robert's breaths became shallower and his body functions slowed down, Jane stood by his bed and stated, "I love you, and with my whole heart I wish you free of this world and free of ALS." Robert died peacefully at home surrounded by his parents, children, and, of course, Jane.

Resources and Organizations with Good Web Sites

National Hospice and Palliative Care Organization: www.nhpco.org
Center to Advance Palliative Care: www.papc.org
Education for Physicians on End-of-Life Care: www.epec.net
Last Acts Palliative Care Task Force Report: www.lastacts.org

Recommended Reading

Hospice and Home Care

Brown, Rebecca. *The Gifts of the Body*. New York: HarperCollins, 1994.

Callanan, Maggie, and Patricia Kelley. *Final Gifts: Understanding the Special Awareness, Needs and Communications of the Dying*. New York: Bantam, 1992.

Duba, Deborah. *Coming Home: A Guide to Dying at Home with Dignity*. New York: Aurora Press, 1987.

Dunn, Hank. *Hard Choices for Loving People: CPR, Artificial Feeding, Comfort Measures Only and the Elderly Patient*. Herndon, VA: A & A Publishers, 1994.

Eidson, Ted (ed.). *The AIDS Caregiver's Handbook*. New York: St. Martin's Press, 1993.

Grollman, Earl (ed.). *Concerning Death: A Practical Guide for the Living*. Boston: Beacon, 1974.

Mace, Nancy L., and Peter V. Rabins. *The 36-Hour Day: A Family Guide to Caring for Persons with Alzheimer's*. Baltimore: Johns Hopkins University Press, 1991.

Saunders, Cicely, M.D., and Mary Baines, M.D. *Living with Dying: The Management of Terminal Disease*. Oxford and New York: Oxford University Press, 1989.

Stoddard, Sandol. *The Hospice Movement: A Better Way to Care for the Dying*. New York: Random House, 1991.

Spiritual Perspectives

Beck, Charlotte Joko. *Nothing Special*. San Francisco: Harper-Collins, 1993.

Chodron, Pema. *Start Where You Are*. Boston: Shambhala, 1994.

Dalai Lama, the Fourteenth. *Kindness, Clarity and Insight*. Ithaca, NY: Snow Lion, 1984.

Dass, Ram, and Paul Gorman. *How Can I Help?* New York: Alfred A. Knopf, 1985.

Dossey, Larry, M.D. *Recovering the Soul: A Scientific and Spiritual Search*. New York: Bantam, 1989.

Fox, Matthew. *A Spirituality Named Compassion*. Harper San Francisco, 1979.

Frankl, Viktor. *Man's Search for Meaning*. New York: Simon & Schuster, 1959.

French, R.M. (trans.). *The Way of a Pilgrim and The Pilgrim Continues His Way*. Harper San Francisco, 1965.

Goldberg, Rabbi Chaim Binyamin. *Mourning in Halachah*. Brooklyn, NY: Mesorah Publications, 1991.

Harrison, Gavin. *In the Lap of the Buddha*. Boston: Shambhala, 1994.

Hellwig, Monika. *What Are They Saying About Death and Christian Hope?* New York: Paulist Press, 1978.

Jampolsky, Gerald, M.D. *Good-bye to Guilt: Releasing Fear through Forgiveness*. New York: Bantam, 1985.

Kabat-Zinn, Jon. *Wherever You Go, There You Are: Mindfulness Meditation in Everyday Life*. New York: Hyperion, 1993.

Khenpo, Nyoshul. *Natural Great Perfection*. Ithaca, NY: Snow Lion, 1995.

Khyentse, Dilgo. *The Wish-Fulfilling Jewel: The Practice of Guru Yoga According to the Longchen Nyingtig Tradition*. Boston: Shambhala, 1988.

Krishnamurti, J. *Think on These Things*. New York: Harper & Row, 1964.

Kushner, Harold. *When Bad Things Happen to Good People*. New York: Schocken, 1981.

Levine, Stephen. *Who Dies? An Investigation of Conscious Living and Conscious Dying.* New York: Doubleday, 1982.

May, Gerald, M.D. *The Awakened Heart: Living Beyond Addiction.* San Francisco: HarperCollins, 1991.

Merton, Thomas. *Contemplative Prayer.* New York: Doubleday, 1969.

Nhat Hanh, Thich. *Being Peace.* Berkeley: Parallax Press, 1987.

Pastoral Care of the Sick. New York: Catholic Book Publishing Co., 1983.

Riemer, Jack (ed.). *Jewish Reflections on Death.* New York: Schocken, 1974.

Steindl-Rast, Brother David. *A Listening Heart: The Art of Contemplative Living.* New York: Crossroads, 1983.

Suzuki, Shunryu. *Zen Mind, Beginner's Mind.* New York: Weatherhill, 1970.

Teresa, Mother. *A Simple Path.* New York: Ballantine, 1995.

Theophan, Sr., the Recluse. *The Path of Prayer.* Newbury, MA: Praxis Institute Press, 1992.

Trungpa, Chogyam. *Training the Mind and Cultivating Loving-Kindness.* Boston: Shambhala, 1993.

Wilber, Ken. *Grace and Grit: Spirituality and Healing in the Life and Death of Treya Killam Wilber.* Boston: Shambhala, 1991.

Dying and Death

Bryan, Jessica (ed.). *Love Is Ageless – Stories About Alzheimer's Disease.* Felton, CA: Lompico Creek Press, 2001.

Callahan, Daniel. *The Troubled Dream of Life: Living with Mortality.* New York: Simon & Schuster, 1993.

DeSpelder, Lynne Ann, and Albert Lee Strickland (eds.). *The Path Ahead: Readings in Death and Dying.* Mountain View, CA: Mayfield, 1995.

Jury, Mark and Dan. *Gramps: A Man Ages and Dies.* New York: Penguin, 1976.

Kavanaugh, Robert. *Facing Death.* New York: Penguin, 1972.

Krauss, Pesach. *Why Me? Coping with Grief, Loss, and Change.* New York: Bantam, 1988.

Kubler-Ross, Elisabeth. *On Death and Dying.* New York: Macmillan, 1969.

Longaker, Christine. *Facing Death and Finding Hope*. New York: Broadway Books, 2001.

Lund, Doris. *Eric*. Philadelphia: J.B. Lippincott, 1974.

Ruskin, Cindy. *The Quilt: Stories from the Names Project*. New York: Pocket Books, 1988.

Tolstoy, Leo. *The Death of Ivan Ilych*. New York: Penguin, 1960.

Buddhist Teachings on Death and Dying

Chagdud Tulku Rinpoche. *Life in Relation to Death*. Cottage Grove, OR: Padma Publishing, 1987.

Fremantle, Francesca, and Chogyam Trungpa (trans.). *The Tibetan Book of the Dead*. Boston: Shambhala, 1975.

Kapleau, Philip (ed.). *The Wheel of Death: A Collection of Writings from Zen Buddhist and Other Sources on Death, Rebirth, Dying*. New York: Harper & Row, 1971.

Mullin, Glenn H. *Death and Dying: The Tibetan Tradition*. Boston: Arkana, 1986.

Rangdrol, Tsele Natsok. *The Mirror of Mindfulness: The Cycle of the Four Bardos*. Boston: Shambhala, 1987.

Rinpoche, Sogyal. *The Tibetan Book of Living and Dying*. San Francisco: HarperCollins, 1992.

Bereavement

Caine, Lynn. *Widow*. New York: William Morrow, 1974.

Froman, Paul Kent. *After You Say Goodbye: When Someone You Love Dies of AIDS*. San Francisco: Chronicle Books, 1992.

Gilbert, Kathleen R., and Laura S. Smart. *Coping with Infant or Fetal Loss: The Couple's Healing Process*. New York: Bruner-Mazel, 1992.

Guest, Judith. *Ordinary People*. New York: Viking, 1976.

Lewis, C.S. *A Grief Observed*. New York: Bantam, 1963.

Lukas, Christopher, and Henry Seiden. *Silent Grief: Living in the Wake of Suicide*. New York: Bantam, 1987.

Murray Parkes, Colin, and Robert Weiss. *Recovering from Bereavement.* New York: Basic Books, 1983.

Sarnoff Schiff, Harriet. *The Bereaved Parent.* New York: Viking Penguin, 1977.

Stillion, Judith M., Eugene E. McDowell, and Jacque H. May. *Suicide Across the Life Span: Premature Exits.* New York: Hemisphere, 1989.

Tatelbaum, Judy. *The Courage to Grieve: Creative Living, Recovery and Growth through Grief.* New York: Harper & Row, 1980.

Volkan, Vamik D., and Elizabeth Zintl. *Life after Loss: The Lessons of Grief.* New York: Collier, 1994.

SECTION 3

Resources

CHAPTER 13

Finding a Cure and Improving Living with ALS

How the ALS Association Helps Patients and Families

Mary Lyon

About the ALS Association

The mission of the ALS Association (ALSA) is to discover the cause and cure for *amyotrophic lateral sclerosis* (also called *ALS* or *Lou Gehrig's disease*) through dedicated research, and improving the lives of people

> The mission of the ALS Association (ALSA) is to discover the cause and cure for amyotrophic lateral sclerosis.

with the disease. This mission is addressed by providing patient support, information/education for health care professionals and the general public, and advocacy for regulatory and legislative issues. To improve systems for clinical care, ALSA is an important partner in the multidisciplinary team approach to the clinical management of ALS.

What Does ALSA Do?

Research: Working to Find the Cause, Cure, and Treatment for ALS

The ALS Association has an organized program of scientific research that includes encouraging, identifying, funding, and monitoring relevant, cutting-edge research into the cause, means of prevention, and possible cure for ALS. Over the past 10 years, the ALSA has funded $25 million in ALS research—$12.5 million in just the last 3 years. Through an application and review process that is patterned after the National Institutes of Health's (NIH) rigorous process, abstracts and proposals are peer-reviewed and ranked by ALSA's Scientific Review Committee, consisting of renowned neuroscientists. Each year over 200 abstracts for scientific study are submitted for consideration.

The ALSA's Research Program is dedicated solely to ALS-specific research. Hallmarks of the program include:

- An emphasis on inclusiveness and partnerships.
- Research projects in partnership with the NIH, Centers for Disease Control (CDC), Department of Defense (DOD), pharmaceutical and biotechnology companies, and other ALS organizations.
- Extensive and broad portfolio of international research projects that are investigating over 100 diverse scientific issues.
- Research covering every scientific hypothesis of the cause of ALS.
- The ALSA-initiated projects come from new discoveries and questions, and are funded in a fast-track manner with review and advice of a blue-ribbon panel of scientific reviewers.
- Both basic science and therapeutic trials of drugs and other treatments in animals and humans are sponsored by ALSA.
- A prestigious postdoctoral fellowship sponsored by ALSA assures that top young investigators are supported in their interest in ALS research.

ALSA conducts scientific workshops that bring together ALS researchers and non-ALS investigators renowned in their respective specialties to explore specific ALS-relevant topics such as Inflammation and

ALS, Environmental Factors and Genetic Susceptibility, and Young Investigator's Workshops.

Clinical Management Research Grant Program

The purpose of this research program is to stimulate and support studies that will help patients deal with the symptoms of ALS and improve the quality of their lives. Examples of funded projects include an evaluation of the effects of exercise in people with ALS and a study to determine if beginning noninvasive ventilation earlier in the disease will prolong and improve quality of life. The ALSA has funded 13 projects with over $250,000.

Patient Services: Providing Information, Care, Support, and Services to Patients and Families

Feelings of hope, a positive mental attitude, and knowledge are powerful weapons in the battle against ALS. The ALSA's information materials and

> Feelings of hope, a positive mental attitude, and knowledge are powerful weapons in the battle against ALS.

services are designed to offer hope, give needed information about living with ALS, and encourage people to live their lives to the fullest.

The generosity of ALSA's donors assures that all patient and family services and materials are provided without charge. Information from the ALS C.A.R.E. database in North America indicates that ALSA is the not-for-profit, voluntary ALS health organization that is most frequently cited as the most valuable source of information for people with ALS. The Association works to provide timely and authoritative information on the research, clinical, and advocacy issues that are important in the fight against ALS. The Association offers the following resources and information:

Toll-free Information and Referral Service

Patients and family members can dial (800) 782-4747 and be connected to informed, caring people who will answer questions, mail literature about ALS, and offer hope and support.

Mail

The Information and Referral Service is also available by e-mail, fax, or letter.

Web Site

ALSA's Web site (www.alsa.org) includes information about the disease, resources for clinical care and second opinions, and how to get more information. Printed materials are reproduced on ALSA's Web site.

Manuals

A very popular source of information for patients and families are ALSA's *Living with ALS* manuals—a set of six paperback books designed to take the patient through each of the stages of ALS, offering ways to cope and therapies to treat many of the symptoms of ALS. Manuals are provided without charge to patients and families, and can be ordered by calling the toll-free number or writing to ALSA by U.S. mail or e-mail. The ALS Association's *Living With ALS* manuals are also available for reading and printing on the Web site. Manual topics include:

- *What's It All About*
- *Coping with Change*
- *Managing Your Symptoms and Treatment*
- *Functioning When Your Mobility Is Affected*
- *Adjusting to Swallowing and Speaking Difficulties*
- *Adapting to Breathing Changes*

Videos

The ALSA is pleased to offer a series of four videos that are companion pieces to the *Living with ALS* manuals. They can be ordered, free of charge, by telephone, e-mail, or from the Web site. The topics include:

- Mobility, Activities of Daily Living, and Home Adaptations
- Swallowing Problems and Feeding Tubes
- Breathing Problems and Use of Noninvasive Ventilation
- Communication Solutions and Symptom Management

Another video that is available is a physician roundtable discussion of the clinical management practice guideline recommendations, which resulted from the American Academy of Neurology's review of the available clinical research results.

FYI Information Index

A series of brief flyers on over 40 specific topics is available, including swallowing tips, minimizing fatigue, and speech devices. Topics are listed in the Library section on the Web site.

Research News

New research grants awarded by ALSA are published twice a year. Chapter and support group newsletters keep patients aware of breaking news from the research front. Bulletins on research findings are posted on the Web site home page. Anyone can sign up for the "Keep Me Informed" service and receive e-mails of all ALS Association news releases.

Clinical Drug Trials and Drug Development Update

Information on drug trials and where they are being conducted—as well as what is new in the development of drugs for ALS—are included in the *Drug Development Update*, available in print and on the ALSA Web site.

Recommended Reading and Videos

A suggested reading list can be sent to patients on request; ALSA's library includes a variety of videos that are provided to patients.

ALSA Center Certification Program

The ALSA developed standards for ALS clinics in collaboration with medical experts to encourage quality care that is interdisciplinary and that includes doctors who are knowledgeable and experienced in making the diagnosis and taking care of people with ALS. Clinics that pass the rigorous application and site visit reviews are certified as ALSA Centers. It is ALSA's intent that the 2-year recertification requirement helps to improve the quality of the ALSA Centers. Another benefit of the ALSA Center Program is the facilitation and fostering of information exchange among the medical directors and staff of the ALSA Centers. A list of current certified ALSA Centers is on the Web site. There were nineteen ALSA Centers as of December 2003.

Standards and Requirements:
- Active support for the ALS clinic from the local ALSA chapter or free standing support group
- An existing multidisciplinary and interdisciplinary ALS clinic
- A clinic director with well-recognized expertise in ALS
- Full availability of neurologic diagnostic and other necessary medical services
- A number of established ALS patients seen and a pattern of new ALS patients added to those being seen, sufficient to justify ALSA Center status

Someone to Talk to
Sometimes people with ALS, their families, and caregivers just need someone to talk to—a person who will listen to them and understand the day-to-day challenges they are facing. ALSA provides telephone contact with concerned, knowledgeable people from both the National Office and each ALSA chapter.

Patient and Family Education Programs
Many ALSA chapters sponsor patient/family education programs covering general information about ALS as well as specific tips and hints that make living with this disease easier. Check with your local chapter of ALSA for their "Ask The Experts" conference schedule.

Support Groups
Talking with other people who are living the same experience can help decrease the common feelings of depression and isolation. ALSA's chapters and freestanding support groups conduct hundreds of support group meet-

ings across the country every month. Support groups range from an informal sharing of successful ideas of how to solve problems of daily living to formal medical presentations. There are support groups for newly diagnosed patients, caregivers and—in some areas—children of people with ALS. In all cases, the emphasis is on helping people maximize their physical functioning and maintain quality in their lives.

Equipment and Speech Device Loan Program
ALSA chapters provide equipment on loan to patients for use in the activities of daily living, including wheelchairs, walkers, and bedside commodes. Many chapters also have a variety of augmentative-alternative communication devices that are made available to patients.

Respite Programs
Family caregivers have demanding and often overwhelming jobs. A break from caregiving to go shopping, see a movie, or spend a day with friends can provide a needed change and rest. Many ALSA chapters offer reimbursement for respite care for families to help them cope with the demands and challenges of caring for a loved one with ALS.

Transportation Program
Patients who require sophisticated wheelchairs and modified vans may need more help getting from home to an ALSA Center or to support group meetings than family and friends can provide. Some chapters are able to offer transportation services to patients.

Caregiver Support
The ALSA recognizes the need of caregivers to have information and support. ALSA reaches out to help and support caregivers through the information and referral services provided by the national office and local chapters, the Web site, literature, support groups, and respite programs.

Patient Bill of Rights for People with ALS
When people are knowledgeable about their rights regarding health care, they are more likely to get the services and care they need. ALSA's *Patient*

Bill of Rights for People with ALS (Table 13-1) is an information and advocacy tool for patients and families as they negotiate the health care system.

Home Visits and Care Management
Many local chapters of ALSA provide home visits and care management to the ALS families in their service area.

Support, Information, Recommendations, and Referrals
Support, information, recommendations, and referrals for palliative care are provided by ALSA.

TABLE 13-1

The Amyotrophic Lateral Sclerosis Association's Patient Bill of Rights for People Living with ALS

As a person living with ALS, you have the right to:

1. Receive comprehensive information about ALS, including treatment options and resources for your health care needs. This includes the right to communicate with your government representatives regarding policies of the FDA, NIH, and other agencies that relate to ALS.

2. Participate in decisions about your health care with the highest level of decision-making possible. This includes the right to discontinue or refuse treatments and therapy.

3. Receive ALS specialty care in a timely manner.

4. Receive health care that is coordinated and individualized for you across the spectrum of home, hospice, hospital, nursing home, outpatient, and workplace, and throughout all the phases of your illness.

5. Access health care benefit coverage and life insurance coverage without discrimination based on your ALS diagnosis or disability.

6. Obtain clear, timely information regarding your health plan, including benefits, exclusions, and appeal procedures.

7. Review your medical records and have the information in your records explained to you.

8. Prepare an advance directive in order to state your wishes regarding emergency and end-of-life treatment choices.

9. Receive care that is considerate, respects your dignity, and holds information confidential. You have this right no matter what choices you make about treatments and therapy, what your disabilities related to ALS might be, or what your financial circumstances are.

10. Receive maximum support to enhance the quality of your life and have your family involved in all aspects of your health care.

ALSA as Advocate: Creating Changes at the Local, State, and Federal Levels to Benefit People with ALS

The ALS Association advocates on behalf of ALS patients through its year-round, nationwide advocacy program, centered in its Capitol Office in Washington, DC. The overall goal is to advocate for public policy in support of ALS research and ALS-related health issues, including increased funding for NIH research on ALS, accelerated treatment development, and access to proper care and treatment. Led by ALSA, advocacy efforts of the ALS community resulted in significant changes in Social Security, which now waives the 2-year waiting period for disability and Medicare to begin, streamlines the process for review of ALS disability applications, and provides presumptive disability for people applying for Supplemental Security Income. If you want more information about ALSA's Advocacy Program or to get involved, contact the Advocacy Office in Washington, D.C. (see "Where to Get Help," page 194).

Raising Awareness: Increasing Public Knowledge about ALS to Foster More Research and Services

Raising general awareness about ALS will lead to an increase in research funding and support for clinical and support services. Everyone has a part to play in increasing ALS awareness—from talking with community friends and neighbors to writing a letter to the editor of a local newspaper. ALSA's National Office leads a public awareness campaign that includes articles, features, and public service announcements in major newspapers and magazines, and on radio and television. Although the awareness campaign is yearlong, special emphasis is given to events in May, which has been designated "National ALS Awareness Month." ALSA's national publication is distributed to more than 120,000 people and includes reports on ALSA's programs, services, research findings, clinical trials, and programs for patients. Contact ALSA to be added to the mailing list.

ALSA strives to involve and engage patients and families in the process of raising awareness and advocating for legislative changes. A broad base of committed people in communities across the country can create a powerful voice for increasing research funding and improving care and treatment.

Other Ways ALSA Advances the ALS Cause

Since the mid-1990s, ALSA representatives have met with scientists from the pharmaceutical industry who have or who are currently developing ALS drugs. Several companies participate in the *Drug Company Working Group*, which was first established to encourage combination medication therapy. Recently, the meetings have expanded into ALS workshops that bring together researchers, physicians, representatives from the Food and Drug Administration (FDA) and NIH, and industry representatives to discuss the newest research and incentives for treatment development for people with ALS.

Representatives of ALSA regularly attend scientific and neurologic professional meetings to keep abreast of the most current research and treatment news, and raise awareness about ALS by sponsoring exhibit booths. ALSA staff routinely participate in the annual meetings of the American Academy of Neurology, American Neurological Association, and the Society for Neuroscience as a continuing means to promote ALS research and ALSA's national patient services programs. These national meetings provide opportunities to publicize ALSA's scientific and clinical management research grant programs, as well as the services the organization provides to ALS patients and their families.

ALSA sponsors three special activities every year: a day of ALS legislative advocacy in Washington, DC; a conference for ALSA's voluntary and staff leadership; and an ALS Clinical Conference for nurses, social workers, and therapists who work with ALS patients.

ALSA provides financial and human resources to support many ALS professional activities, such as the International Symposium of ALS/MND and the ALS Clinical, Assessment, Research, and Education (ALS C.A.R.E.) program—a North American database intended to improve care for people with ALS.

The ALS Association maintains communication and working relationships with federal and private agencies. Examples include the FDA,

NIH, CDC, DOD, Veterans Affairs (VA), Social Security Administration (SSA), Health Care Financing Administration (HCFA—Medicare), National Health Council (NHC), and the Paralyzed Veterans of America (PVA). Efforts with these groups are directed toward creating changes and making improvements that benefit people with ALS.

You Are Not Alone: The Story of Jim and Peg

Jim began noticing weakness in his right hand at age 52, when he and his wife, Peg, started redecorating their home. The youngest of their three children had just moved out, and Jim and Peg were looking forward to more time to themselves, a vacation, and fresh paint and carpet for the house. It was not until 8 months later that Jim learned he had ALS. By then, his right hand was very weak, and Jim could tell that his arm was beginning to be affected too.

Within days of learning that Jim had ALS, Peg began to search the Internet looking for answers and help. She found the ALS Association's Web site with a wealth of information and resources. Later, Peg said that one of the best things she did was sign up for "Keep Me Informed," a free e-mail update service provide by ALSA. The steady stream of e-mail updates she received about research and other advances in ALS proved to be one of the lifelines to hope for their entire family.

Peg reached out via the ALS Association's Information and Referral Service's toll-free number and learned about the importance of a second opinion for Jim. She was excited to learn about several clinical drug trials being conducted and was hopeful that Jim might be qualified to enroll in one soon. With the clinical trials contact information right on the Web site, Jim and Peg spent the afternoon reviewing the information and contacting study coordinators.

The ALS Association's Information and Referral Service encouraged Peg and Jim to contact the chapter in their community for local services and direct support. They began attending the chapter's monthly support group, where the emphasis was living with ALS. Although they were reluctant to go to the first meeting, Peg and Jim were pleasantly surprised at the warmth, hugs, and laughter with which so many people greeted them. At the chapter's Walk to D'Feet ALS®, all three of their children were there with their friends to walk in support of "Jim's Team" to raise awareness and money for ALS research and services.

Through the chapter, Jim learned about the local certified ALSA Center, where his care was personalized and all of the multidisciplinary team members were experienced and knowledgeable about ALS. There was an atmosphere of hope and a positive approach to helping Jim cope with his symptoms so that he could maintain as much of his ability to function as possible. The ALSA Center had a number of research projects in progress, and Jim enrolled in one of the clinical trials.

Jim was outspoken by nature and wanted to make a difference for himself and others with ALS. He found a perfect way to express this through the ALSA's Advocacy Program. As chair of his chapter's Advocacy Committee, Jim talked with local and state legislators about living with ALS and what was needed to improve life for people with this disease and their families. He traveled to Washington, DC, and participated in the annual Advocacy Day, visiting his members of Congress to advocate help for people living with ALS.

Patient services representatives from the chapter made a series of home visits to help Jim and Peg arrange for several changes in their home to allow Jim mobility and function throughout their house. Jim found that he could no longer perform his work as a graphic artist, so he and Peg were relieved to learn that advocacy efforts were successful in making important changes in the Social Security Administration regulations that would make benefits easier and quicker to get. The ALS Association's *Living with ALS* series of manuals and videos proved to be valuable tools that they used over and over. Jim and Peg particularly appreciated that so many patients and their families spoke from their experiences and their hearts in the videos.

As time went on, Jim needed a number of pieces of equipment and he was able to borrow them from his local chapter. The equipment helped him stay mobile, independent, and active. Peg was grateful for the difference the equipment (such as lift devices) made for her as Jim's caregiver. Peg found that she and Jim got a great deal of comfort and support from the chapter staff and volunteers. Their help and advice throughout their journey with ALS was reassuring and comforting to them and their children.

Peg became the primary caregiver as Jim's disease progressed. The chapter respite program helped Peg have time away from her responsibilities as Jim's caregiver to do simple errands, visit friends and family, and attend special occasions. During a home visit by a chapter staff member, both Jim and Peg remarked that throughout their battle with ALS, they felt they were part of a team or family of people from the ALS community and that the chapter had supported them and been there every step of the way.

Help for the Person Who Is Newly Diagnosd with ALS

The diagnosis of ALS is a life-changing event for the individual with the disease and his loved ones. Understandably, the diagnosis is inevitably met by an overwhelming sense of fear, worry, and loss. With the help of several families who have first-hand experience of what those first few months were like, ALSA developed the following suggestions for how to get the information and help you need:

1. *Get a second opinion.* Refer to the related article and FYI reference materials on the ALSA's Web site.
2. *Educate yourself about ALS and how to live with the disease:*
    (a) As of December 2003, there is one FDA-approved drug for the treatment of ALS: Rilutek®. It is modestly effective; other treatments are being evaluated in clinical trials on an ongoing basis.
    (b) Avoid getting too much information about issues and decisions you may not need to face or that may be far into the future.
    (c) Look for reputable, authoritative sources of information.
    (d) Contact the ALSA's National Office or your local chapter for information and for quality resources for further materials and information.
    (e) Review the ALSA's Web site and focus on information useful to you in the first several months after diagnosis.

(f) Refer to the FYI on the Web site titled *How to be a Careful Internet User* to guide you in selecting quality sources of information.

(g) Beware of the unsubstantiated claims regarding "too good to be true" treatments and cures that abound on the Internet.

(h) Ask the ALSA for a copy of the *Patient's Bill of Rights for People with ALS*, which is a useful self-advocacy tool (see Table 13.1, page 186).

3. *Tell the news.* This can be an especially difficult thing to do. Who to tell, when to tell, and how to tell others about your diagnosis are some of the things to consider. The ALS Association offers some tools to help explain ALS to children. Staff can also help you think about and decide who to tell, when, and how.

4. *Learn about opportunities to participate in a clinical trial.* Clinical studies to evaluate the safety and potential benefit of various treatments for ALS are an option to consider. Information about current clinical trials can be found in the Research section on the ALSA Web site.

5. *Find out about current research and sign up for "Keep Me Informed" on ALSA's Web site to learn about research news when it is released.* The Research section of the ALSA's Web site provides an excellent overview of ALS research and news releases.

6. *Become informed about benefits including disability, health care, and financial issues.* Depending on how ALS is affecting you, you may be considering stopping work, or you may plan to work for a considerably longer time. Each person has her own individual situation. In either case, it can be useful to learn about benefits you may need at a later time. Become familiar with the Americans with Disabilities Act to know your rights in the community and in the workplace. Additional resources regarding information about benefits can be found in the Internet and Agency Resource list at the end of this chapter.

7. *Find the resources and services that can help you now and in the future.*

(a) The ALSA chapters and the National Office have resource and referral information that can help you identify useful resources.

(b)   An ALS Clinic with an experienced ALS physician and multi-disciplinary team may be available in your community or within travel distance. If not, find a physician who is knowledgeable about ALS and in whom you have confidence. The ALS Association's Web site includes listings of the certified ALSA Centers, ALS Clinics that work with local chapters, and ALS physicians nationwide.

(c)   Obtain a copy of the *ALS Practice Parameter*, which is a set of recommendations for medical care in five aspects of clinical care.

(d)   Many local communities and states have programs and services such as financial help, respite care, and equipment loan that can help ALS families.

(e)   You may be eligible for benefits if you are a veteran. Contact the ALSA or the Paralyzed Veterans of America for more information. See the FYI on *Veterans Benefits* on the ALSA's Web site.

8.   *Adjusting and coping.* The diagnosis of ALS is a significant change, and it is natural to have feelings of depression, anger, anxiety, loss, and/or sadness. These can be dealt with in a number of ways:

(a)   Consider talking with your physician or a counselor about your feelings.

(b)   Take medications to help with the psychological symptoms common in many people with ALS.

(c)   Consider the benefits of attending a support group (face-to-face or on the Internet) to talk with others who have gone through what you are experiencing. They can offer ideas that help.

(d)   There are several Internet bulletin boards and chat rooms that many people with ALS find helpful.

(e)   Talk with your loved ones about your feelings and ask for their support.

9.   *Consider becoming active in ALSA's Advocacy Program.* Your involvement can give a voice to your feelings and needs, and can truly make a difference for people with ALS. Contact the Advocacy Office of the ALSA.

Where to Get Help

The ALS Association:

National Office
27001 Agoura Road, Suite 150
Calabasas Hills, CA 91301-5104
(800) 782-4747 toll-free Information and Referral Service for patients and
    families
(818) 880-9007 business number
(818) 880-9006 facsimile
www.alsa.org—Web site
alsinfo@alsa-national.org—e-mail Information and Referral Service for
    patients and families
Advocacy Office
(202) 638-6997 business telephone
(202) 638-6316 business fax
39 Chapters (http://www.alsa.org/serving/chapter.cfm)
12 Freestanding Support Groups
19 certified ALSA Centers (http://www.alsa.org/serving/category.cfm#centers)

Internet and Agency Resources

Internet Chat Rooms

- http://groups.yahoo.com/group/living-with-als/chat
- http://clubs.yahoo.com/clubs/alsormnd
- http://rideforlife.com/als66
- http://neuro-mancer.mgh.harvard.edu/cgi-bin/Ultimate.cgi?action=
  intro&category=2&BypassCookie=true
- ALS Digest—To subscribe, please e-mail Bob Broedel at bro@met.fsu.edu
- Patients Bill of Rights—http://www.alsa.org/als/rights.cfm
- Aids to Daily Living—http://www.alsa.org/resources/product.cfm
- Informative Links—http://www.alsa.org/resources/friends.cfm
- Caregiving—http://www.alsa.org/resources/friends.cfm#caregiving
- Research—http://www.alsa.org/research/

- Physicians List—http://www.alsa.org/resources/physician.cfm
- Government Agencies —http://www.alsa.org/resources/friends.cfm#gov
- Americans with Disabilities Act—http://www.ada.gov
- The ACCESS Program—A toll-free resource knowledgeable about Social Security Disability and Supplemental Security Income. Phone Toll Free: (888)700-7010
- The Social Security Administration—http://www.ssa.gov
- Medicare—Toll Free: (800) MEDICARE. Web Address: http://www.medicare.gov
- Paralyzed Veterans of America—http://www.pva.org

For specific information and resources regarding the items discussed in this chapter, contact the ALSA and the other organizations listed. By becoming informed, prepared, and involved, you and your loved ones can use the information and resources as tools to help you fight ALS and maintain quality of life. You are not alone. The ALS Association is here to help.

The ALSA is the only not-for-profit voluntary health agency in the United States dedicated solely to amyotrophic lateral sclerosis. Having a single focus ensures that all of ALSA's resources are directed exclusively to ALS. The vast majority of ALSA's funds go for research (53 percent) and patient services/community services (16 percent), while only 6 percent of expenses were allocated for administrative costs in 2002.

The people who provide leadership for ALSA by serving as members of the National and Chapter Boards of Trustees are volunteers whose personal lives have been touched in some way by ALS. Working diligently to make scientific discoveries and improve the lives of people living with ALS, ALSA is committed to engaging patients and families in the process of setting and achieving organizational goals. ALSA has volunteers and paid staff at the National Office; most of the chapters have full-time patient services staff.

The ALS Association is fortunate to have physicians, nurses, and other medical professionals who graciously serve as voluntary members of ALSA's Medical Advisory Committee. The purpose of the Medical Advisory Committee is to provide ALSA with information and advice on clinical and research issues of importance.

CHAPTER 14

The Muscular Dystrophy Association (MDA), ALS Division

Ronald J. Schenkenberger

The Muscular Dystrophy Association's ALS Division offers a comprehensive range of services to people and families coping with amyotrophic lateral sclerosis (ALS). The ALS Division has been at the forefront of the scientific battle against the disease since Eleanor Gehrig, Lou Gehrig's widow, served as an early volunteer leader of the Association in the 1950s. MDA has continued its leadership role in ALS research and services and, in 2004, the Association will spend $15.6 million on its ALS program.

MDA works aggressively through its worldwide research program to find effective treatments and a cure. MDA also provides practical help for the everyday needs of those with ALS. The medical care, assistive devices,

> The Muscular Dystrophy Association nurtures the spirit as well as the body.

information, services, and support provided by MDA nurture the spirit as well as the body, assuring individuals and families that they are not alone in their journey but are part of a caring community united in the fight against ALS.

Clinics: A Full Range of Medical Care

The Association maintains approximately 230 hospital-affiliated clinics, located in every state. MDA clinics provide diagnostic services and follow-up care to people with ALS, as well as those affected by any of the more than forty other neuromuscular diseases under MDA's umbrella.

In addition, as of the end of 2003, there were thirty MDA/ALS Research and Clinical Centers at major medical institutions across the country. These centers are directed by many of the nation's leading ALS specialists: neurologists who are conducting ALS research and have the latest information on medically managing the disease.

Anywhere across the country, people with ALS can go to an MDA clinic or an MDA/ALS Center and receive diagnostic and follow-up care, including referrals and prescriptions for a full range of therapies and equipment.

MDA's ALS Centers utilize a team approach to medical care, allowing patients and their caregivers to see all of the necessary specialists in one visit. Besides physicians, the team typically includes such skilled professionals as speech, respiratory, physical, and occupational therapists; and rehabilitation specialists, social workers, and genetic counselors. Referrals can be made to pulmonologists, cardiologists, or gastroenterologists as needed. Those who attend the clinic may also receive consultations and prescriptions for wheelchairs and other orthopedic equipment, flu shots, training in basic daily care techniques, and more.

An MDA staff representative—usually a Health Care Service Coordinator (HCSC) from one of MDA's over 200 local offices—attends every clinic session and serves as an ongoing link between patients and medical staff. The HCSC also coordinates many nonmedical services for those with ALS, including support groups, educational conferences and seminars, and the provision of assistive equipment from MDA loan closets at no charge.

Initial Diagnosis

The only requirement for receiving an evaluation at an MDA clinic or MDA/ALS Center is the written recommendation of a physician in whose judgment a person may have ALS. If the disease diagnosed is not ALS or one of the other forty-plus diseases covered by MDA, appropriate referrals will be made to the health agency or community agency covering the specific illness diagnosed. A physician's statement of diagnosis is kept on file with the Association to ensure the person's eligibility for MDA services.

Payment for Authorized Medical Services

It is the policy of MDA to assist with payment for those services authorized in its program that are not covered by private or public insurance plans or other community resources. These payments are made directly to the institution in which the MDA clinic is located or to authorized vendors. Association policy requires that only MDA may place orders and make payments.

MDA Support

MDA clinics offer an interdisciplinary team approach to initial diagnosis and follow-up care. Individuals suspected by their physicians of having ALS or one of the other neuromuscular disorders included in MDA's pro-

> MDA clinics offer an interdisciplinary team approach to initial diagnosis and follow-up care.

gram have access to a nationwide network of hospital-affiliated MDA clinics staffed by neuromuscular disease specialists. The MDA clinic team can advise patients and their families about the initial diagnosis and recommend measures to medically manage ALS. MDA clinic follow-up care ranges from management of symptoms to medical intervention designed to assist individuals in maintaining the highest possible quality of life.

Diagnostic Exam

The first step in medical care is determining the nature of the disease. The MDA clinic team can perform diagnostic examinations and recommend pertinent laboratory tests. Some of these tests may be extensive, yet in most instances, they can be done on an outpatient basis. Information about genetically based diagnostic testing is available at the MDA clinic. Following clinical examination and analysis of the laboratory tests, many neuromuscular diseases can be quickly and accurately diagnosed. Some neuromuscular diseases may require a differential diagnosis. The first question the physician will seek to answer in performing a diagnosis is whether muscle function is abnormal because there is a disease of muscle itself, or whether muscle function is abnormal because of a disorder that has developed in other tissue (e.g., nerve, as in the case of ALS).

Follow-Up Medical Care: Managing ALS

Upon diagnosis, a number of services may be recommended by the MDA clinic team as measures to medically manage ALS.

Periodic Reevaluations

Follow-up visits are usually scheduled quarterly, but at certain stages in the progression of the disease, more frequent checkups may be indicated.

Physical, Occupational, Respiratory, and Speech Therapy

An MDA clinic physician may prescribe physical, occupational, respiratory, and/or speech therapy to be administered by a certified practitioner as part of a treatment program. Therapy may be offered at the MDA clinic, at another facility, or in the home.

Physical Therapy

MDA will assist with the payment for one consultation annually to (a) evaluate the need for physical therapy, and (b) instruct family members and others on how to administer prescribed exercises. Physical therapy can neither arrest the disease process nor restore affected muscle tissue; however, it may help keep still healthy muscles functioning and may delay the onset of contractures.

Occupational Therapy

MDA will assist with payment for one consultation annually as prescribed to enable people to make maximum use of their physical capabilities by being instructed in the use of specially designed assistive devices and daily living aids in their home and work environments.

Respiratory Therapy

MDA will assist with payment for one consultation annually as prescribed for instruction in the use of prescribed respiratory therapy equipment designed to augment or increase vital lung capacity.

Speech Therapy

When prescribed by an MDA clinic physician, the Association will assist with payment for one consultation annually to evaluate the muscles responsible for speech and swallowing. A speech-language pathologist can determine if the use of a communication device and/or modifications to meals are appropriate.

Social Services

Social services are a vital aspect of the MDA clinic program; they are a resource for families seeking direction in identifying alternative sources of payment for medical services.

Cooperation with Primary Care Physicians

A summary report may be made available upon request to the person's primary care physician after the initial clinic examination and after each re-evaluation. In addition, MDA clinic directors may advise your other specialty physicians on problems related to specific conditions.

Genetic Counseling

Genetic counseling is available to the families of those who are affected by an inherited form of ALS.

Flu Inoculations

Influenza may be particularly hazardous to people with ALS. Flu inoculations are arranged by MDA when medically prescribed.

Transportation

MDA will assist in arranging for transportation to appointments at the nearest MDA clinic in those instances when family or community resources are not available.

Direct Services

Services to enhance mobility and independent living are available in each community through MDA's local network of chapters and field offices.

Wheelchairs/Leg Braces/Communication Devices

When medically prescribed by the local MDA clinic physician, MDA assists with the purchase of wheelchairs, leg braces, and communication devices, regardless of age, education, or employment status. The maximum allowable amount of financial assistance toward the purchase of a wheelchair, leg braces, or a communication device is established by MDA annually.

Recycled Equipment

MDA provides, to the extent feasible and when available, recycled wheelchairs and other durable medical equipment in good condition when medically prescribed. Families are encouraged to return equipment to MDA for use by others when the individual for whom it was prescribed no longer needs the equipment. MDA accepts recycled durable medical equipment at its local chapters and field offices.

Repairs/Modifications

The Association assists with payment toward the cost of repairs/modifications to all wheelchairs and leg braces routinely authorized for MDA payment. The amount allowable toward repairs/modifications is established by the Association annually.

Accessibility and Awareness

MDA actively monitors and supports programs and legislation relevant to people with disabilities, such as medical care, insurance, accessibility, transportation, education, independent living, and personal assistance services.

Community Resources

Services not provided by MDA are often available from other community agencies. MDA assists in securing help from these community resources.

Support: Emotional, Practical, and Physical

The psychological distress of ALS can threaten an individual's well-being almost as much as the physical effects. The MDA watchword is: "Help for today and hope for tomorrow."

Support is a critical component of MDA's mission and it is expressed through such avenues as professionally facilitated support group meetings, hosted Internet chats, and public information campaigns that raise awareness about ALS.

In many cities across the country, MDA offers ALS support groups where people with ALS, caregivers, and other family members can meet and talk with those who have been down the same road. People with ALS and professional facilitators share the kind of practical advice, emotional support, and humor that makes coping easier.

For those who do not have access to a meeting or who are not the "support group type," there are several weekly MDA Internet chats specifically for people with ALS and their families. They are hosted by people with ALS or ALS caregivers and offer a place to vent, question, share, inform, joke, and socialize from the comfort of home. In addition, special chats focusing on the health care aspects of ALS are led by expert physicians, researchers, and therapists year-round.

Research: A Worldwide Quest

In 2003, MDA awarded some $7.7 million in research grants to fund approximately seventy-five ALS research projects around the world. In addition to probing the mystery of why nerve cells die, researchers test drugs and compounds that may slow progression or more effectively manage symptoms. MDA-funded scientists are investigating genetic factors in ALS, the Gulf War connection, stem cell therapy, autoimmune factors, potential use of drugs for breast cancer and arthritis in ALS, the development of a "drug cocktail" to treat ALS, and many other avenues.

MDA researchers were instrumental in the development of riluzole (Rilutek®), the only currently FDA-approved drug treatment for ALS. MDA's ALS Division supports an ongoing search for other drugs to slow the progress of the disease.

Among the promising clinical trials launched in 2004 is one involving minocycline, a medication used to treat bacterial infections that slowed ALS deterioration in animal studies. Building on a small trial that showed the drug to be safe for use with ALS patients, MDA is supporting a 13-month, 400-person trial at 24 sites.

People with ALS are invited to participate in MDA-sponsored and other clinical trials for which they qualify. Up-to-date information on trials can be found through MDA's ALS Web site and its monthly newsletter, as well as through the physicians at MDA/ALS Centers and clinics.

MDA's Translational Research Advisory Committee (TRAC) was formed in 2002 to help navigate the increasingly difficult regulatory path from promising lab results to available drugs or therapy—"from bench to bedside." The committee is made up of experts in basic and clinical research, and drug development in industry and government policy. It reflects MDA's commitment to work closely with industry and government to speed potential treatments to those who need them.

In June 2003, MDA, the National Institutes of Health (NIH), and several pharmaceutical companies sponsored a conference of 100 ALS experts in Tarrytown, NY titled *ALS Clinical Trials: The Challenge of the Next Century*. In addition to reviewing the current status of ongoing trials, the group decided to hold regular meetings with the aim of improving trial designs, and to take steps toward training clinical investigators and encouraging rapid research in all areas that might lead to clinical trials in ALS.

MDA Is There Every Step of the Way

The underlying message MDA emphasizes to those with ALS is: "As you face your life with ALS, remember you, too, are not alone. MDA has served people with ALS for more than 50 years and will be there for as long as it takes to defeat this deadly foe."

Allen's Story

Allen Roberts* had never heard of ALS and was only vaguely aware of the term "Lou Gehrig's disease." The name "MDA" also held little meaning for him, beyond his having sometimes watched MDA's Telethon on Labor Day weekend.

But when Allen was 47, he started inexplicably tripping over curbs and the steps to his office. His leg muscles began to do an odd twitching dance. He fell flat on his face while playing golf. Urged on by his wife, Diane, Allen sought a medical explanation for his confusing symptoms. After conducting some research of his own, he suspected ALS, but he wanted to be sure.

After fruitless months of bouncing from doctor to doctor, Allen heard from a friend that MDA included ALS in its program. He contacted the

---

*Allen Roberts is a fictional person based on the case histories of several people with ALS served by MDA.

closest MDA office, which then referred him to a local MDA clinic and the nearest MDA/ALS Center. He ultimately found himself signing in at an MDA/ALS Center at a major medical school near his hometown, armed with a list of questions, a lot of frustration, and not a little fear.

After an extensive examination and testing, Allen was told he had ALS. Doctors and staff at the center explained what the disease was and described the services that MDA provided.

The expert health professionals at the MDA/ALS Center were able to answer the questions that were troubling Allen after offering him the latest diagnostic tests and taking a history. They emphasized the hope offered by current research and explained that life expectancy for those with ALS was steadily increasing, thanks to current treatments and technology.

Once Allen received his diagnosis of ALS, his thoughts turned to finding a cure or effective treatment to help him retain his strength for as long as possible and adapt to the changes ALS was causing in his body. The medical professionals at the MDA/ALS Center prescribed Rilutek®, which is most effective when begun early in the course of the disease. They also advised him on other strength-preserving techniques. MDA gave him information on research and clinical trials, and he took steps to participate in a trial near his home.

Although Allen still was walking at the time he received his ALS diagnosis, he soon began to fall more frequently and often had trouble getting back up. Diane worried about leaving him alone, and the couple learned through MDA about many techniques and devices that could help him at various stages of ALS.

Now that his condition had a name and its effects were progressing, Allen needed a steady stream of up-to-date information to make informed choices, maximize his health, and maintain a sense of control. He turned to the ALS Division of MDA for its monthly newsletter, extensive Web site, care guides, videos, books, and local seminars.

He began to visit some of the ALS online chat sessions and offered to be interviewed by local media during ALS Awareness Month in May. He also appeared on the local broadcast of the annual Jerry Lewis MDA Telethon to share his experience with the community.

As the disease progressed, Allen and Diane became regular participants at a local MDA support group for families affected by ALS. They found new strength and understanding encouragement from friends they made there.

Allen felt that MDA's public information campaign on ALS—including television and newspaper public service announcements—helped to decrease some of the isolation of having a rare disease, and it aided advocacy efforts for improved governmental benefits and more federal research dollars.

In a heartbeat, Allen Roberts went from blissful ignorance of ALS to devastating awareness. But thanks to his own courage, the love of family and friends, and the services, support, and hope provided by MDA, he has moved beyond devastation. Although his life has changed radically, he is quick to point out that it is still a very good life. And, with MDA's extensive support, he knows he is not alone.

Resources

Muscular Dystrophy Association
ALS Division
3300 E. Sunrise Drive
Tucson, AZ 85718
(800) 572-1717
(520) 529-2000
www.als.mdausa.org

Web Site and Local Information

The ALS Web site at www.als.mdausa.org provides general information about ALS, late-breaking news and current information about research and clinical trials, transcripts of online chats with ALS experts, "Ask the Experts" answers to the questions of ALS patients; information on obtaining ALS publications and video resources, downloadable ALS publications, a listing of MDA/ALS Centers, and current and back issues of *The MDA/ALS Newsletter.*

To locate the nearest MDA office for information about local programs, look under "Muscular Dystrophy Association" in the telephone book, call (800) 572-1717, or send an e-mail to mda@mdausa.org. You also can go to www.mdausa.org/locate/index.html and enter your zip code.

MDA has more than 200 local offices that can provide referrals to clinics and information about support groups, equipment loan closets, volunteering opportunities, and other local programs. Local offices also organize conferences and seminars on ALS led by expert health care providers and scientists.

A schedule of chats on the Internet for people with ALS and their families can be found at this Web site: www.mdausa.org/chat/calendar.html.

Information about ALS clinical trials can be found at this Web site: www.mdausa.org/research/ctrials.html.

Another MDA Web site, MDA en Español, provides current information about ALS and other diseases in MDA's program in Spanish at www.mdaenespanol.org. Publications in Spanish also are available on this site.

MDA Publications

MDA publications and videos are available through local offices or the national office.

The *MDA/ALS Newsletter* is published monthly and mailed without charge to people with ALS who are registered with MDA. The newsletter offers user-friendly information about the latest research findings, conference reports, clinical trials, caregiver resources, as well as profiles of people with the disease and their activities and accomplishments, contact information about useful programs, and legislative/governmental news relevant to people with ALS.

MDA's bimonthly magazine *Quest* is mailed without charge to people with neuromuscular diseases, including ALS, who are registered with MDA. The award-winning magazine features a blend of scientific, practical, and supportive articles on a variety of topics related to living with neuromuscular diseases.

MDA books and booklets about ALS are regularly revised to feature the most current information:

- *101 Hints to "Help-with-Ease" for Patients with Neuromuscular Disease* (in English and Spanish)
- *ALS: Maintaining Mobility*
- *ALS: Maintaining Nutrition*
- *Facts about Amyotrophic Lateral Sclerosis* (in English and Spanish)
- *Meals* (a cookbook of easy-to-swallow foods)
- *When a Loved One Has ALS: A Caregiver's Guide*

MDA Videos

- *ALS Update*
- *ALS: Maintaining a Positive Perspective*
- *Breath of Life*
- *Breathe Easy*
- *The MDA Support Group and You*
- *With Strength and Courage: Understanding and Living with ALS*

CHAPTER 15

Negotiating the Insurance Maze

With Dorothy E. Northrop, MSW, ACSW

This chapter provides a simple, useful overview of the different kinds of insurance and lessens the occurrence of any surprises. We hope that you will use it as a tool for financial and life planning to manage the impact of ALS on you and your family. We urge you to begin this planning *now*, before you absolutely need to act on the information. This chapter will serve as a guide to the questions that you need to ask.

A diagnosis of ALS brings the need for insurance into sharp focus. Most people look at insurance as a necessary evil that they pay a lot of

> A diagnosis of ALS brings the need for insurance into sharp focus.

money for over a long period of time in the event that they will need to use it some time in the distant future. Most do not really understand how insurance works, and they are often overwhelmed by insurance language when they try to educate themselves. But, however challenging such writing may seem, you *can* understand the benefits that you are entitled to—in return for all those years you saved for a rainy day by paying insurance premiums and Social Security/FICA taxes. Of course, you will probably always wish the benefits were better. You will often be surprised by what insurance does not cover, but you will be equally surprised at just how much insurance *does* cover.

There are two broad categories of insurance, one that provides income protection when you cannot work as a result of illness, and one for the payment of health care costs. The social worker at your ALS clinic or health care facility may be able to help you understand these general concepts. However, variations in coverage are huge, and you are advised to get specific information from your benefits administrator, insurance broker, and applicable state and federal agencies.

Income Protection

A diagnosis of ALS does not mean that you should immediately stop working; however, it is a good time to begin explorations with your workplace human resources department and/or union to find out what benefits you may be entitled to. Find out whether your workplace provides either short- or long-term disability plans. You should discuss filing for disability with your physician when you feel that the overall cost to your well-being of working outweighs its many benefits.

Short-Term Disability

Short-term disability plans are usually group policies offered by an employer that provide partial income replacement for a period of 6 months to 2 years. These plans are sometimes mandated by the state (often referred to as *State Disability*) and are funded through payroll deductions. Currently, New York, New Jersey, California, Rhode Island, Hawaii, and Puerto Rico have this type of mandated insurance. If your company is headquartered in a state other than the one you work in, you should make sure that the benefits quoted to you are the ones for the state in which you pay taxes.

Long-Term Disability

Employer-sponsored long-term disability policies are sometimes paid for by employers but more often they are paid for by the employee. Such policies vary widely and you should thoroughly investigate your coverage with both human resources and the company issuing the policy. If you have purchased an individual disability policy, find out how the coverage is activated and the benefits paid. Talk with your doctor, nurse, and social worker about assisting with the inquiry, or consider legal counsel if you are having problems getting the carrier to take your inquiries seriously.

If you are employed by a company that has a group disability insurance plan for its employees, or belong to any professional or fraternal organization that offers this coverage, you should check to see if you are eligible. You may automatically be entitled to the basic amount of disability insurance that is offered to the entire group by virtue of your membership in one of these groups, regardless of your ALS diagnosis or other medical history. This basic coverage is called *guaranteed-issue coverage*. Your ALS diagnosis will probably prevent you from buying coverage over and above this basic amount, but you should still be assured of some basic coverage. Since organizations may offer this type of group coverage only as a one-time incentive for membership, one strategy is to join as many organizations as you can that offer this type of group disability coverage. These multiple group memberships would thus enable you to piece together adequate coverage. It is certainly in your best interest to obtain disability coverage while you are actively working; it is virtually impossible to obtain disability coverage once a person leaves work due to disability.

Social Security

The Social Security Administration (SSA) pays three types of benefits: Social Security Retirement, which is based on having paid the required Federal Income Contribution Act (FICA) taxes as a worker and reaching retirement age; Social Security Disability Income (SSDI) which is based on having paid FICA taxes and being disabled; and Supplemental Security Income (SSI), which is based on financial need regardless of what a worker has paid into the Social Security system.

Social Security Disability Insurance

You can qualify for the Social Security Disability Insurance (SSDI) program if you are a legal resident, have paid (FICA) taxes, and have worked recently and long enough.

When you are working and paying Social Security taxes, you earn credit every time you earn $890 (2003 figures) over the course of a calendar year. You will have earned four credits for the year when you have earned $3,560. You may earn up to but not more than four credits in a year. Age at the time of application will determine the number of credits needed, but if you are 31 years or older, you must have earned at least 20 credits in the 10 years immediately before you became disabled. Younger people require fewer credits, but they still need at least six.

Information about the credits required to qualify can be obtained from the Social Security Administration's Disability booklet or www.socialsecurity.gov. To do adequate financial planning, you should determine if you qualify for the program at the earliest possible opportunity.

The SSA made qualifying for SSDI much easier for people with ALS in August 2003. With appropriate medical evidence to support the diagnosis of ALS, the SSA will qualify the applicant as disabled without proof of substantial physical impairment. Occasionally, employees at Social Security may not be aware of the new ruling, but you can direct them to amendments 404 and 416 of Title 20 of the Code of Federal Regulations.

You should apply for benefits as soon as you can no longer work because there is a 5-month waiting period from the date you are deemed disabled by the SSA before you can receive benefits. SSA will ask for names, addresses, and phone numbers for all of your doctors; dates of treatment; your work history for the past 15 years; and your most recent W-2 form. If you encounter any difficulties, have an unusual situation, or have questions that SSA cannot answer satisfactorily, the A.C.C.E.S.S. (Advocating for Chronic Conditions, Entitlements and Social Services) Program (1-888-700-7010) may be able to help.

Check with Social Security to see if any of your family members are eligible for benefits as well. If so, you will be asked to provide their birth certificates and Social Security numbers. Assembling all these documents early will make the process less painful when you apply.

Social Security Income

Social Security Income (SSI) is funded through general tax revenues and is not based on work history, but rather on financial need. People who qualify for SSI usually also qualify for food stamps and the health insurance program Medicaid (see page 224). You can get more information at your local Social Security office by calling 1-800-772-1213, and from www.ssa.gov.

Health Insurance

There are more than a dozen different types or "categories" of health insurance plans and a tremendous number of variations among plans within each category. Fortunately, three very simple distinctions take us a long way toward understanding health insurance options. They are the *government* plans: Medicare and Medicaid; group or individual indemnity, or *fee-for-service* plans; or *managed care* plans (HMO, EPO, PPO, POS). Virtually any plan you select will reflect some combination of these—for example, a government-provided group managed care plan or a private, fee-for-service plan, purchased on an individual basis.

Employer-sponsored Group Programs

When an employer sponsors a health plan, the coverage is called a *group* plan. These plans often offer wide coverage at a lower rate than individual plans. These plans cover more people and "spread the risk," in that some people in the plan will use a lot of services while others will use very few.

In general, if you are covered under a fee-for-service plan, you may use the services of any appropriately credentialed physician or allied health provider you wish. To the extent that you use *covered* services—that is, services that are eligible for coverage under your particular contract, and so long as you meet all of the policy and procedural requirements for using such a service, your plan will either pay a specific sum (a part or the total cost of your care) to your provider or reimburse some or all of your costs directly to you if you pay the provider. The exact amount that you will be reimbursed depends on the terms of the insurance contract, but it is typically a percentage (70 to 80 percent) of the "usual, customary, and reasonable" cost. This cost is determined by insurance companies and reflects their calculation of the standard amount charged by the same type of providers for the same service in the same community.

Managed care is a system of organizing health care that integrates the financing and delivery of health care to covered individuals through arrangements with selected providers. These providers are available to furnish a relatively comprehensive array of health services, although many plans lack or limit coverage for durable medical equipment, such as wheelchairs, or for care in the home. Explicit standards are used by the managed care organization to select health care providers and equipment vendors for participation in the plan. Formal policies and procedures exist for ongoing quality assurance and utilization review in the provision of care to enrolled individuals. There are generally significant financial incentives for enrollees to use providers and procedures associated with the plan, rather than using *out-of-plan* providers.

The most common and best-known form of managed care is the *health maintenance organization*, or *HMO*. In return for a fixed, periodic payment, HMO providers offer a wide range of health care services, including preventive care. The HMO may have a single central facility, several branch sites, or may exist as an array of individual providers and facility locations that have contracted to provide service for the HMO. Two common forms of HMO are the *staff model*, in which physicians and other providers are employees of the HMO; and the *individual practice association*, or *IPA*, in which physicians and other providers maintain their personal practices but agree to serve as HMO providers under the terms of the HMO when caring for an HMO enrollee. In the traditional HMO, an enrollee who goes out-of-plan does not receive coverage or reimbursement for those outside services, except in special cases such as emergencies.

The second most common managed care arrangement is the *preferred provider organization*, or *PPO*. In this arrangement, physicians and other providers contract with the PPO sponsor to reduce their fees when a member of the PPO comes to them for service. Plan members choosing to use out-of-plan providers receive some coverage, but less than if they had used one of the preferred providers.

An increasingly popular hybrid, aimed at controlling costs while retaining consumer choice of providers, is the *point-of-service HMO*. Combining aspects of HMOs and PPOs, the point-of-service plan functions as an HMO, but provides limited (70 to 80 percent of the total charge) coverage for out-of-plan providers. Thus, a person who chooses to consult an out-of-plan provider will generally receive coverage, but less than if he had stayed within the HMO for that care. Point-of-service premiums are higher than HMO premiums.

How Do Managed Care Plans Work for Someone with ALS?

Managed care organizations work the same way for people with ALS as they do for other enrollees. However, some studies and individual anecdotes raise some concerns. These concerns relate primarily to the inadequacy of access to ALS specialists. For example, the managed care organization may have very few (or no) neurologists or other health care providers who are expert in caring for people with ALS, or they may have such specialists, but the enrollee can only receive a referral to one if the primary care provider—generally a family physician or internist—chooses to make the referral. Because the managed care organization places great emphasis on saving money, the primary care physician may have major financial or other incentives to limit referrals to specialists.

Informal surveys suggest that ALS enrollees who have adequate access to ALS specialists are generally pleased with their managed care experience. They are usually dissatisfied with the managed care organization when they have inadequate access. PPOs try to address this problem by offering some coverage for out-of-plan consultations or treatment, but they are often more costly than HMOs. Point-of-service HMOs attempt to address this problem by combining the key features of HMOs (comprehensive care and low cost) with that of PPOs (covered access to out-of-plan providers, although typically at higher cost than staying in-plan).

In short, people with ALS may fare well in managed care organizations—especially point-of-service HMOs—if the plan they choose is a comprehensive one and, most important, provides ready access to ALS specialists. During open enrollment periods, when considering a managed care plan, make sure to ask about access to providers with expertise in ALS care and about coverage for the kinds of equipment or home care that are sometimes needed by a person with ALS.

Extending Health Insurance Coverage after You Stop Working

Health benefit provisions in the Consolidated Omnibus Budget Reconciliation Act of 1985 (COBRA) are designed, in part, to ensure that people who lose employment-related group health insurance benefits because of job termination or reduction in job hours will be able to maintain group coverage for themselves and their families for limited periods of time. If you and other members of your family are covered under a group health plan through your employer, each covered member may be able to buy the same coverage at a slightly higher premium for 18 months and possibly as long as 36 months following termination of employment. However, the employer no longer contributes to the premium, and the full cost of coverage becomes the responsibility of the employee.

The law generally covers group health plans maintained by employers with twenty or more employees. It applies to plans in the private sector as well as those sponsored by state and local governments. COBRA does not apply to plans sponsored by the federal government, certain church-related organizations, or to companies with fewer than twenty employees. If you work for one of these organizations, you will need to research and get advice about your options. Many states have *mini-COBRA* laws that provide continuation protection for those employed in businesses with less than twenty employees. However, this protection is often not as generous as the federal legislation.

A COBRA plan can be terminated if the employer discontinues group health coverage, the employee-paid premium for continuation of coverage is not paid on time, the covered member becomes entitled to Medicare, or a covered member obtains coverage from another employer plan (you will need to find out if there is a pre-existing condition exclusion period).

Although people with ALS may qualify for Medicare, family members who are covered under your plan may qualify for COBRA coverage for up to 36 months. Ask the employee benefits manager at your company about COBRA and read the plan booklet. There are very strict deadlines for notifying your health plan administrator if you are electing initial coverage and when the Social Security Administration makes its determination for disability for extended coverage. Make sure that you understand the rules and adhere to the requirements to avoid accidentally missing a deadline and losing coverage.

Companies that are not subject to COBRA may offer a standard conversion to another health plan. This coverage will generally be less comprehensive than in the employer group plan and will likely cost more than the premium charged within the group.

Medicare

Medicare is a federal health insurance program that covers people over the age of 65 and many disabled people under the age of 65. If you are enti-

> Medicare is a federal health insurance program that covers people over the age of 65 and many disabled people under the age of 65.

tled to Social Security Retirement or SSDI benefits, you are also eligible for Medicare. Disabled people generally need to wait 24 months after receiving SSDI benefits to become eligible for Medicare. The Benefits Improvement Act, enacted in 2001, waived the 2-year waiting period for people with a diagnosis of ALS so that they become eligible when they begin receiving SSDI. Those people who receive SSI only are not eligible for Medicare.

Some public employees and clergy are exempt from Social Security taxes because they have paid into a separate retirement system and, thus, they are not eligible for Social Security benefits. However, many of these employees have paid Medicare taxes. Other individuals qualify for Social Security and Medicare through their spouse's work history. Some people may have elected to retire early and receive Social Security, but were subsequently diagnosed with ALS before age 65. If you are in these categories, we strongly encourage you to contact your employer, Social Security office (800-722-1213), and Medicare (800-633-4227) to determine your benefits.

Part A of Medicare covers hospital, qualified skilled nursing home stays, and home care. If you are eligible for Medicare, you cannot decline Part A coverage. Part B coverage charges a monthly premium and covers outpatient hospital care, doctor's fees, diagnostic tests, durable medical equipment, ambulance service, and many supplies. Part B can be declined, but we recommend carrying this coverage as it is used extensively by people with ALS.

Medicare has many advantages. You can go to any physician or certified home care agency or equipment vendor that accepts Medicare. Everyone knows what will be covered and not covered and—with a few exceptions—there is no prior authorization process.

Medicare's disadvantage is that it only covers 80 percent of your costs and historically has not covered prescription medication. The Medicare Prescription Drug Improvement and Modernization Act of 2003 will begin to give Medicare recipients some cost relief for their prescriptions (see Medicare Prescription Benefit below). Some insurance policies are either canceled or become supplemental "Medigap" policies (see below) when Medicare becomes effective. It is advised that you know what will happen to your current insurance policy *before* you become eligible for Medicare. Counseling is available through your state health insurance counseling program (SHIP). Contact Eldercare at 1-800-677-1116 if you need help locating your local program.

Medicare Supplement (or "Medigap") Plans

Medicare pays a large part (generally 80 percent) of the health care costs for those covered, but the insured individual remains responsible for Medicare deductibles and coinsurance, and for services and excess provider charges not covered under Medicare. These additional costs can be substantial. To cover these unpaid costs, many private insurers offer Medicare Supplement (also called "Medigap") plans to supplement Medicare services and to cover Medicare beneficiary costs (the other 20 percent).

Initially, there was a bewildering array of Medigap plans on the market and many questionable marketing practices, such as companies selling several overlapping plans to the same individual. To address these problems, the National Association of Insurance Commissioners developed ten standardized Medigap plans, called "A," "B," "C," and so on, through plan "J." While each plan differs in the specific coverage offered, a given plan is always the same wherever it is sold in the United States. Thus, if you purchase plan B in New York, it will be identical to a plan B purchased in California, Nebraska, or elsewhere. However, it is important to note, that individual companies charge different amounts for the same plan. Thus, insurance company X may charge substantially more for plan B than insurance company Y does for an identical plan B. So it pays to shop around. Medigap plans must accept all people over age 65, regardless of pre-existing conditions. However, there are no federal regulations requiring that Medigap plans cover those under 65 who receive Medicare with Social Security Disability benefits. Therefore, states differ in the Medigap plans that are available to SSDI recipients. Not all standardized plans are offered in every region of the country. Your local SHIP office can help ascertain what is available where you live.

Many Medicare recipients will opt for a *managed Medicare* plan to fill their Medigap needs. Be aware that when signing on for *managed*

> Be aware that when signing on for *managed Medicare,* you are signing over your long awaited Medicare benefits to a private insurance company to manage.

Medicare, you are signing over your long awaited Medicare benefits to a private insurance company to manage. You are required to follow all the rules of the HMO/PPO to get coverage for health care costs (see description of HMO and PPO plans on pages 215–217), but the company should cover everything that Medicare covers. The main disadvantage of these policies is your loss of choice as to which doctors (including ALS specialists), equipment vendors, and home care agencies you can use. Most referrals to doctors and for equipment will have to go through what can be a lengthy prior authorization process. The main advantages to these plans are lower premiums and sometimes medication coverage. Often medications are *capped* or limited to approximately $1,000 per year, often with only generic medication coverage. Many medications have no generic equivalent because they are still protected under patent laws and, therefore, will not be covered. You must weigh the benefits of lower premiums with managed care plans against the cost of decreased choice.

Medicare Working with Other Health Plans

When you become eligible for Medicare due to disability, your individual plan coverage (a plan that you pay for yourself—not employer-sponsored) cannot be canceled. Some people with employer-sponsored insurance are able to maintain their health plan without buying COBRA. You may be eligible for health coverage through your spouse, some other organization (union, fraternity organization) plan, or a retirement package. Even though there may be a substantial fee involved, many people continue these coverages rather than purchasing a Medigap policy so that they can take advantage of the better prescription coverage available. You should check with the health plan administrator of the private policy to see how they "coordinate benefits" with Medicare. It will save you much aggravation in the future if you understand which policy is *primary*—meaning it is billed first—and how benefits are coordinated between the two.

When you are covered by more than one type of insurance that covers the same health care expenses, one pays its benefits in full as the primary payer and the others pay a reduced benefit as a secondary or third payer. When the primary payer does not cover a particular service (such as medication coverage or certain types of equipment) but the secondary payer does, the secondary payer will pay up to it's benefit limit as if it were the primary payer.

Before you make a decision to keep or terminate this type of coverage, contact your SHIP for more information about your rights to coverage and coordination of benefits between your individual or group coverage and Medicare.

The Medicare Prescription Benefit

The first phase of the program begins in June 2004 with the use of Medicare-approved drug discount cards. Individuals will be allowed to purchase these cards from private companies for an annual fee of approximately $30. Over seventy companies are offering cards and the cards offered vary by the region you live in. Finding the card that will benefit you most will require some diligence on your part. Some drugs may be cheaper on one plan, but that benefit may be outweighed by the higher cost in the same plan for other drugs you use. The average discount will be from 10 to 30 percent off average retail prices. Do compare savings with retailers that offer discounts without cards such as Costco and other mail order companies. If you have a Managed Medicare plan, Medicaid, military or veterans benefits, you will not have an option to purchase cards.

A few resources may help you decide which card gives you the greatest benefit. You can call Medicare (1-800-MEDICARE) or do a comparison online at www.medicare.gov. You will need to give these sources your income level, zip code, and the drugs that you take, and Medicare will give you a list of cards in your area with comparisons of the discount available. You may also find the worksheets from the American Association of Retired Persons Web site at www.aarp.org/prescriptiondrugs helpful.

If your income is less than $12,569 (or $16,862 for couples), you may be eligible to receive a $600 credit in 2004 and again in 2005 and Medicare will cover the cost of the card enrollment fee.

Beginning in 2006, these discount cards will phase out and the new Medicare benefit will help defray the cost of prescription drugs. For the vast majority of Medicare recipients, there will be an optional $35 a month premium with tiered coinsurance payments. (You pay part and Medicare pays part.) You will pay a $250 deductible and 25 percent of costs between $251 and $2,250. You are responsible for 100 percent of costs for the next $1,500 (between $2,251 and $3,600) and then catastrophic coverage kicks in with only nominal fees for drugs.

Medicaid

Medicaid is a medical assistance program for certain individuals and families with low incomes and assets. In addition to offering comprehensive hospital and medical protection, including prescriptions, Medicaid also provides coverage for an array of long-term care services, including nursing home stays. Far fewer people with ALS are eligible for Medicaid than for Medicare because their family income and assets are usually too high to meet the Medicaid requirements.

Medicaid is a joint program of the federal government and each state government. Although the federal government contributes money to the Medicaid program, each state administers its own Medicaid (in California called *MediCal* and in Tennessee called *Tenncare*) program. Medicaid differs from traditional Medicare in another key respect: Medicaid coverage varies from state to state, except for certain core Medicaid-mandated benefits available in every state's program. Thus, it is important to learn the specifics of Medicaid coverage in your own state even if you think that you may not qualify now. Sometimes, you can "spend down" savings on medical care and qualify at a later date.

Veteran's Administration (VA)

Every veteran should contact the VA to learn details of the benefits available to them. In recent years, many veterans of the Persian Gulf War were diagnosed with ALS. This has led to an increased awareness of the needs of ALS patients, and benefits have been easier for all veterans with ALS to obtain. You may be eligible for service-connected benefits if you can document symptoms of muscle weakness within 2 years of active duty, and you may still be eligible for some veteran's benefits including medication coverage even if your disability is nonservice connected. This will be an important benefit if you are receiving Medicare, as Medicare will only cover a portion of your prescription bills. This system can take some time to negotiate if you have never used it before, so it is recommended that you start early in your disease process, even if you do not feel that you need to use their services. You may qualify for category 4 benefits (catastrophically disabled) as your disability increases, which includes equipment and funding for home care and home modifications. ALS is considered under the VA system to be a spinal cord injury or disease that entitles you to work with the Paralyzed Veterans of America. Call them at 1-800-424-8200 to see if they can help you with your disability rating and benefits.

It is important that you register with the VA Health System by completing an enrollment form and submitting your DD214 or honorable discharge certificate. You can contact them at the Enrollment Center at 1-877-222-VETS. You will need a copy of all your medical reports to prove you have ALS. You should make an appointment with a primary care physician and ask for referrals to a neurologist *and* a physiatrist (rehabilitation doctor) to maximize your access to rehabilitation benefits.

Coverage of Treatments for ALS, Including Rilutek®

Here, as in other insurance matters, plans vary greatly in their coverage. In the end, you must investigate coverage under any plan you have or are considering. Most private insurance plans cover the disease-modifying agents that have been approved by the FDA for treatment of ALS as part of their prescription drug coverage provisions. A few do not. Among those that do cover drugs, coverage varies greatly, and coinsurance and copays have been increasing. Many impose deductibles (generally modest ones), coinsurance (ranging from nominal, e.g., $5, to substantial, e.g., 30 percent of the total yearly cost), and/or yearly caps on the total amount they will pay (for example, $2,000/year). They may require submission of documentation of *medical necessity* from your neurologist and then undertake a prior authorization review. Some plans may require that you purchase the medications at designated pharmacies.

The Patient Assistance Program for Rilutek® is administered through the National Organization for Rare Disorders (NORD). This is a program of last resort and will only consider those with no prescription coverage from any source. The application is lengthy and asks for detailed financial information. You can contact NORD at 1-800-459-7599 for more details.

Regarding coverage of other new ALS treatments, nearly all insurers require that a treatment has been approved for prescription use by the U.S. FDA before it will even consider paying for it. A drug that has not been FDA-approved will likely not be covered. Even if a drug is FDA-approved, it may only be approved for particular uses or patients. If you do not meet the criterion, you may not be able to obtain coverage for the drug, even if your insurer covers the drug for plan enrollees who do meet the FDA approval criterion. Coverage for an FDA-approved drug can also be denied if it is being prescribed *off-label* (i.e., to treat a condition not included on the FDA label or package insert).

People participating in clinical trials of an experimental treatment may receive coverage through the research administrators or clinicians conducting the trials. If you are considering entering a trial, ask if you will have to pay some or all of the cost of the experimental agent(s) or any specialized care you will receive.

Long-Term Care Policies

Long-term care policies are beginning to be purchased with greater frequency. They are designed to provide benefits that are not traditionally

> Long-term care policies are beginning to be purchased with greater frequency.

covered in regular health care plans. Typically, they will pay for custodial or attendant care in the home or in an outside facility.

Most people who have these policies are reluctant to activate them too soon for fear they will use up the policy before they really need it. You are encouraged to activate your policy when you begin to need consistent help with your routine activities. Most of these policies have a waiting period during which you are expected to cover the cost of care for a certain period of time—3 to 6 months is common. You should contact your carrier to set up an evaluation with a care/case manager so you can hire someone to assist you and qualify for benefits to which you are entitled. Many of these policies include some coverage for equipment. There will be many items you will need that regular insurance does not pay for that could be covered under this policy. Do not wait before having these items considered.

Life Insurance, Accelerated Death Benefits, and Viatical Settlements

As a part of your financial planning, you should be aware of benefits that may be available to you through your existing life insurance. First, check to see if your policy has provisions to have premiums waived if you are disabled. Second, many people find it preferable to receive money in advance from a policy that they have paid into for a long time in order to pay for needed equipment or care when they need it, rather than accumulating debt. You should begin researching whether your policy has an accelerated death benefit (ADB) provision. The clause will specify the time period for life expectancy (usually 24 months or less) under which the benefit can be activated. The company will then pay generally 50 to 80 percent of the value of the policy in either a lump sum or monthly payments. Some companies will give you a loan against future benefits if no ADB clause exists.

Viatical settlements can be another good way to finance current needs, but you need to do comparison shopping between brokers to secure the best deal. A viatical settlement is a transaction in which a broker buys an insurance policy, passes on to the insured person 50 to 85 percent of its value, and then receives the cash from the policy after you die. This option is one that requires "buyer beware," as there are many scams and bad deals in this industry. If you are considering this option, I strongly recommend reading Cash for the Final Days by Gloria Grening Wolk as a place to begin your research. These options may carry tax consequences and so you should seek guidance from your financial advisor or attorney.

Hospice Coverage

Although many people associate hospice coverage with care at the very end of life, people with ALS should be aware that this coverage can be given for extended periods of time. Most ALS specialists are very aware of exactly what parameters are needed to qualify. Many benefits unavailable under regular health care coverage, such as assistance in the home and medication coverage, are available to hospice patients. All Medicare patients have this benefit, and most private insurances make provisions for this type of care. You should know if these benefits are available to you through your policy and inform your doctor that you will elect this coverage as soon as you are able to qualify.

The Final Word

At times, you will find that your insurance does not pay for things that you think they should. Check with your clinic staff to see if the items denied are typically covered under other patients' insurance. If so, check to see if the class of the item is a covered benefit or not. For example, if your insurance specifically excludes enteral tube feedings, then appealing the decision is fruitless and will only lead to frustration. If the policy covers it with medical justification, ask your doctor or clinic staff to help you write an appeal. It is essential that appeals be written so that you do not get caught in the "he said, she said" world of telephone conversation. If you have thoroughly investigated and know that the benefit is sometimes covered, and if writing an appeal does not work, find out from your state insurance commission how you can appeal beyond the carrier's internal appeal process.

It seems unfair that when you need to concentrate on maintaining your health so often your insurance company feels like an adversary. Let your employer know if you feel that your insurance company is being unreasonable. They have an interest in you receiving what they have invested in. Do not be afraid to ask questions, disagree with decisions, and ask for help. Often, someone who you know will be willing to take on the insurance company with you. The team at an ALS Center can often be helpful. Let them know you need their help.

Resources

Web Sites

- www.alsa.org
  Includes information about ALS, advocacy for patients and families, and support for research.
- www.lougehrigsdisease.net
  Includes information on treatment, causes, equipment, legal and financial matters, and advocacy.
- www.ninds.nih.gov/health_and_medical/disorders/amyotrophiclateral sclerosis_doc.htm
  Amyotrophic Lateral Sclerosis Information Page with information and links about the disease from the National Institute of Neurological Disorders and Stroke.
- www.mdausa.org/disease/als.html
  Includes basic information, articles, clinical trials, and more about ALS for both patients and health professionals. From the Muscular Dystrophy Association.
- www.psigroup.com/ALS.HTM
  A guide to ALS-related information and resources likely to be of interest to medical professionals and/or patients.
- www.alslinks.com/
  Web directory for the ALS community, including organizations, adaptive equipment and apparel, publications, and more.
- www.alsnetwork.com
  Provides a central site for people with ALS to track individual treatment programs and progress while battling ALS.

Products for Patients

- AARP Pharmacy Service: 800-456-2277
  Instant food thickener. Seven days a week 8:00 a.m. to 10:00 p.m., eastern time.
- Bruce Medical Supply: 800-225-8446; fax 781-894-9519
  Instant food thickeners, puree entrees, ready-to-serve thickened juices. Monday through Friday 9:00 a.m. to 8:00 p.m.; Saturday 9:00 a.m. to 5:00 p.m., eastern time.
- Diafoods Thick-it®: 800.647-8170
  Instant food thickener. Call for information for nearest location in your area.
- Graeber's: 800-606-2031
  Instant food thickener and ready-to-serve thickened beverages.
- Med-Diet: 800-633-3438
  Instant food thickeners, puree foods, ready-to-serve thickened beverages.
- Novartis Nutrition Home Delivery Program: 800-828-9194
  Call 24 hours a day, 7 days a week, or order online at www.resource.walgreens.com.
- Tad Enterprises: 800-438-6153
  A line of products for dietary management of dysphagia that includes instant food thickeners, pureed food enhancers, and ready-to-serve thickened juices, milk, and coffee.

Cookbooks and Other Resources

Non-Chew Cookbook by J. Randy Wilson
  Wilson Publishing
  c/o Sandy Olson
  5708 Nicolett Ave. South
  Minneapolis, MN 55419
  1-800-843-2409
  Web site: www.rof.net/yp/randyw
  Sample recipes on Web site

Meals

Available from:
MDA/ALS Clinic
Department of Neurology
6501 Fannin Street NB 302
Houston, TX 77030
Web site: www.bcm.tmc.edu/neurol/struct/als/als5b.html
Sample recipes on Web site

Easy-to-Swallow Easy-to-Chew Cookbook: Over 150 Tasty and Nutritious Recipes for People Who Have Difficulty Swallowing by Donna L. Weihoffen, R.D., M.S., et al.
Available from: www.amazon.com or www.wileyeurope.com/WileyCDA/WileyTitle/ProductCD-0471200743html

The Dysphagia Challenge: Techniques for the Individual, 3rd Edition by Pam Womack R.D., C.D., 1999.
Available by calling: 425-641-4540

Index